The Herbal Body Book

The
Herbal Body
Book

by Jeanne Rose

Illustrations by Michael S. Moore

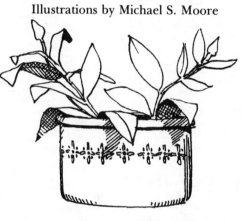

A GD/PERIGEE BOOK

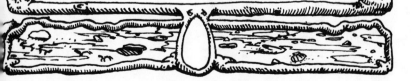

By the same author:
Herbs & Things: Jeanne Rose's Herbal
Jeanne Rose's Herbal Guide to Inner Health

Perigee Books
are published by
The Putnam Publishing Group
200 Madison Avenue
New York, New York 10016

Library of Congress catalog card number: 75-27402
ISBN 0-399-50790-6

First Perigee printing, 1982

Nine previous Grosset & Dunlap printings
Printed in the United States of America

Fourth Impression

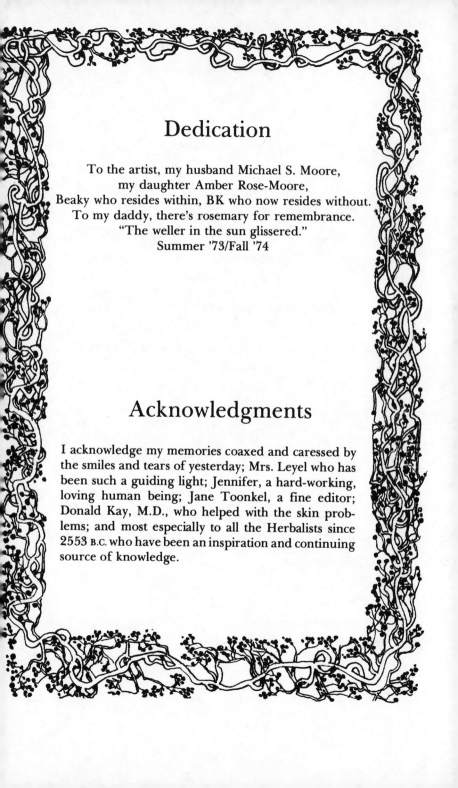

Dedication

To the artist, my husband Michael S. Moore,
my daughter Amber Rose-Moore,
Beaky who resides within, BK who now resides without.
To my daddy, there's rosemary for remembrance.
"The weller in the sun glissered."
Summer '73/Fall '74

Acknowledgments

I acknowledge my memories coaxed and caressed by
the smiles and tears of yesterday; Mrs. Leyel who has
been such a guiding light; Jennifer, a hard-working,
loving human being; Jane Toonkel, a fine editor;
Donald Kay, M.D., who helped with the skin problems; and most especially to all the Herbalists since
2553 B.C. who have been an inspiration and continuing
source of knowledge.

Contents

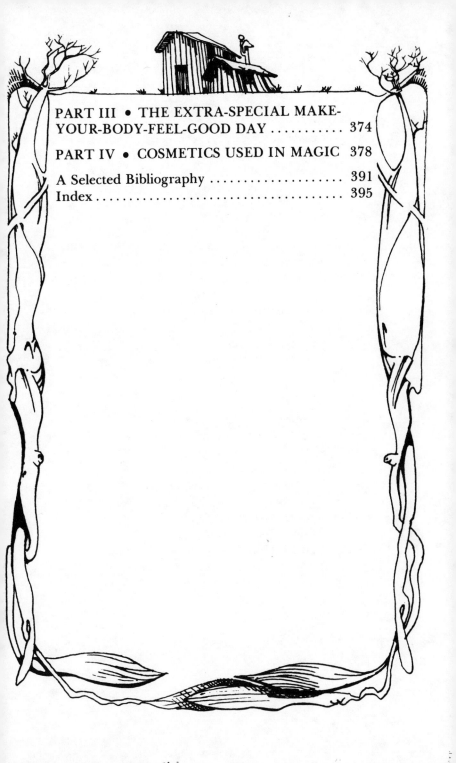

Preface

ABOUT THE PROPOSED JEANNE ROSE HERBALS

The form and scope of the Jeanne Rose Herbals is now defined for the first time. *Herbs & Things* is the first, an herbal primer designed to titillate the general reader with the many subjects that are part of herbal knowledge and tradition, and to excite their attention. The rest of the herbals will take specific parts of this knowledge and enlarge upon them. *The Herbal Body Book* is the second herbal and covers the plants that are used externally for a healthy, natural, and beautiful body. The rest of the herbals will cover many subjects, including Herbal Mother and Child care, Herbs used for Longevity and as Aphrodisiacs, Herbal Animal Care and Human First Aid, Herb Soaps and Massage Oils, and finally, hopefully, Aromatherapy.

Since this particular volume is not a scholarly treatise, botanical names may not be current, but I have made an effort to see that they do agree in at least two or more texts. This information has been obtained from books that are common to most readers and are not necessarily from botanical identification references.

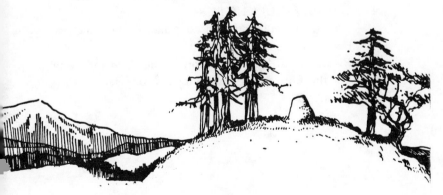

It must be understood that the botanical names listed under each herb do not always refer to one species only, but to others, which in herbal medicine are recognized substitutes.

The line drawings were specially done for this book by my husband, Michael S. Moore, who takes no credit for the front jacket cover.

There are always those who ask me to list the things that I think are most important in life, the things that one must know and do in order to have a healthy, beautiful body and a peaceful mind. If someone were to ask me to now summarize these, I think that I might list the following:

5 STEPS TO HEALTH, BEAUTY AND A PEACEFUL MIND

1. *GOOD NUTRITION*
   For the Cellular Self, also called the Inner Self
2. *EXERCISE*
   For the Muscular Self and to Improve the Circulation
3. *HERBAL HYDROTHERAPY*
   For the Physical Self, also called the Outer Self
4. *MASSAGE*/ACUPUNCTURE
   For the Circulation and to Balance the Electrical Forces in the Body
5. *AROMATHERAPY* (Inhalation for the Mind and Body)
   For the Entire Body and Subconscious Self

Introduction

I sit here on the floor in a house on the island of Oahu and wonder why I am not outside—swimming and surfing or looking through a mask at the beautiful fish. The typewriter hums away in front of me, the trees blow gently outside, the smell of Gardenia, Cup of Gold, Plumeria, and just plain tropical greenness wafts in through the open doors, while the swimming pool of good friend, Dr. Debbie, beckons outside. But I promised to write a book, and a book I will try to type before Beaky appears.

Months later, Michael says that reading my writing is like reading an article originally written in Hindustani for Chinese translated to English by a Japanese, fluent in neither and completely unfamiliar with the subject. Finally Beaky arrives thoroughly complicating matters and further delaying the finish of the book.

Now it is imperative that I teach you how to make the best use of this book. Since it is an herbal book of recipes for beauty and health, decide first what you want to make and for what purpose. Look at Chapter I and decide which herbs to use, then proceed to Chapter III to find out a little bit about the herbs you are going to use (backward to Chapter II if you have to define any words that you may not know), then on to Chapter V or VI to find out where to obtain your desired herbs and finally into Part II to make and cook the desired recipe. Remember that these cosmetics are for women AND men. Please note that my recipes are only suggestions for what you can do; substitute freely with herbs other than those listed in the recipes, for it is only with practice that you will decide exactly what herbs, quantity, and consistency best suit you.

Good Luck!
Jeanne Rose

Publisher's Note

All plants, like all medicines, may be dangerous, particularly to those subject to allergic reactions, if used improperly—if they are taken internally when prescribed for external use, if they are taken in excess, or if they are taken for too long a time. Allergic reactions and unpredictable sensitivities may develop. There are other factors to consider as well: since the strength of wild herbs varies, knowledge of their growing conditions is helpful. Be sure your herbs are fresh and keep conditions of use as sterile as possible.

We do not advocate, endorse, or guarantee the curative effects of any of the substances listed in this book. We have made every effort to see that any botanical that is dangerous or potentially dangerous has been noted as such. When you use herbs, recognize their potency and use them with care. Medical consultation is recommended for those recipes marked as dangerous..

The botanical names listed under each herb do not always refer to one species only, but also to others, which in herbal medicine have been recognized as substitutes.

"Moderation·in all things is all that counts." J. Rose

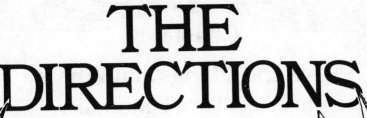

Part I
THE
DIRECTIONS

It is better to prevent than to cure.

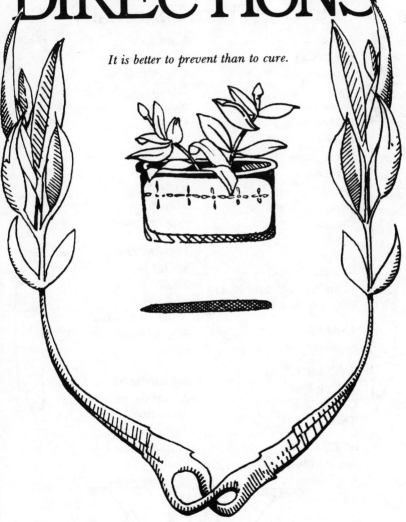

Chapter I

Plants and Things and Where to Use Them Externally

ACNE
Boric Acid
Cantaloupe
Diet
Golden Seal
Herbal Steams
Honey
Horse Bean
Lavender
Mango
Neca 7
Papaya
Sea Salt
Sulfur
Vitamin A Acid
Vitamins A, C, and Niacin
White Willow Bark

Echinacea
Fuchsia Flowers
Gum Benzoin
Myrrh
Noni
Oxalis
Thyme
Tilia

ARM
Mint
Southernwood

ASPIRIN (Salicylic Acid)
Birch Bark
Pansy
Pine Needles
White Willow Bark
Wintergreen
Violet

ANKLES
Southernwood

ANTIBACTERIA
Golden Seal
Orange Peel
Thyme

ASTRINGENT
Agrimony
Alum Root
Bayberry Bark
Bay Laurel
Comfrey Leaf
Comfrey Root

ANTISEPTIC
Bay, California
Bay Laurel

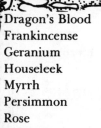

Dragon's Blood
Frankincense
Geranium
Houseleek
Myrrh
Persimmon
Rose
Rosemary
White Oak Bark
Witch Hazel
Yarrow

ATHLETE'S FOOT
Agrimony Foot Bath
Apple Cider Vinegar
Onion Juice
Red Clover
Sage
Soap Bark
Vinegar
Walnut Rind

BEAUTY, GENERAL
Correct Nutrition
Herbal Bath
Herbal Facial
Herbal Steam
Vitamins

BLACKHEADS
Buttermilk
Herbal Steam
Honey Pat
Pansy
Violet

BODY
Alfalfa
Comfrey
Garlic
Parsley
Watercress

BREASTS
Comfrey
Exercise
Lady's Mantle
Quince Seed
Rose Oil Massage
Turnips
Vanilla Oil
Woodruff
Ylang Oil Massage

CELL REGENERATIVE
(see also Rejuvenate)
Comfrey

CELLULITE
Bladderwrack
Broom Flowers
Corn Stigma
Couch Grass Root
Fennel
Greater Celandine
Health Flowers
Horsetail
Jaborandi
Marjoram
Massage

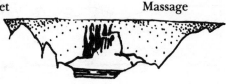

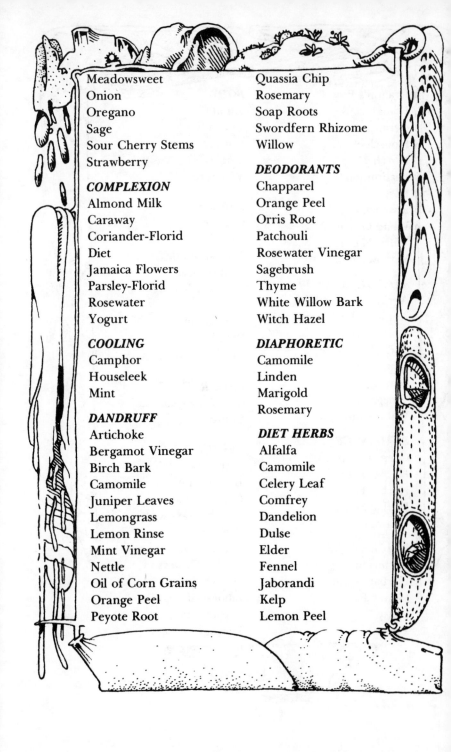

Meadowsweet
Onion
Oregano
Sage
Sour Cherry Stems
Strawberry

COMPLEXION

Almond Milk
Caraway
Coriander-Florid
Diet
Jamaica Flowers
Parsley-Florid
Rosewater
Yogurt

COOLING

Camphor
Houseleek
Mint

DANDRUFF

Artichoke
Bergamot Vinegar
Birch Bark
Camomile
Juniper Leaves
Lemongrass
Lemon Rinse
Mint Vinegar
Nettle
Oil of Corn Grains
Orange Peel
Peyote Root

Quassia Chip
Rosemary
Soap Roots
Swordfern Rhizome
Willow

DEODORANTS

Chapparel
Orange Peel
Orris Root
Patchouli
Rosewater Vinegar
Sagebrush
Thyme
White Willow Bark
Witch Hazel

DIAPHORETIC

Camomile
Linden
Marigold
Rosemary

DIET HERBS

Alfalfa
Camomile
Celery Leaf
Comfrey
Dandelion
Dulse
Elder
Fennel
Jaborandi
Kelp
Lemon Peel

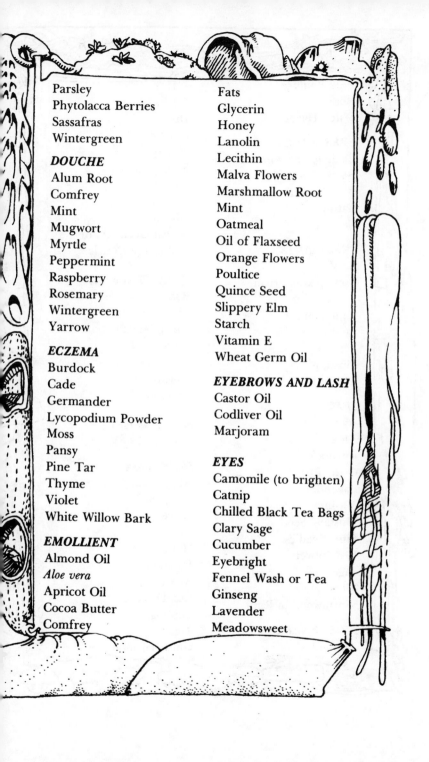

Parsley
Phytolacca Berries
Sassafras
Wintergreen

DOUCHE
Alum Root
Comfrey
Mint
Mugwort
Myrtle
Peppermint
Raspberry
Rosemary
Wintergreen
Yarrow

ECZEMA
Burdock
Cade
Germander
Lycopodium Powder
Moss
Pansy
Pine Tar
Thyme
Violet
White Willow Bark

EMOLLIENT
Almond Oil
Aloe vera
Apricot Oil
Cocoa Butter
Comfrey

Fats
Glycerin
Honey
Lanolin
Lecithin
Malva Flowers
Marshmallow Root
Mint
Oatmeal
Oil of Flaxseed
Orange Flowers
Poultice
Quince Seed
Slippery Elm
Starch
Vitamin E
Wheat Germ Oil

EYEBROWS AND LASH
Castor Oil
Codliver Oil
Marjoram

EYES
Camomile (to brighten)
Catnip
Chilled Black Tea Bags
Clary Sage
Cucumber
Eyebright
Fennel Wash or Tea
Ginseng
Lavender
Meadowsweet

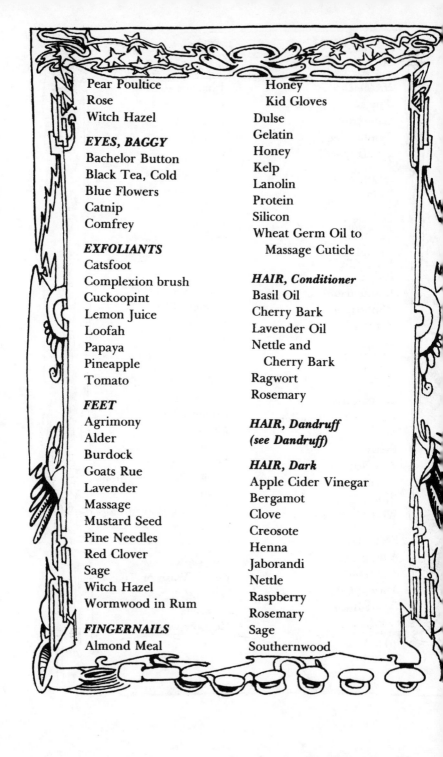

Pear Poultice
Rose
Witch Hazel

EYES, BAGGY
Bachelor Button
Black Tea, Cold
Blue Flowers
Catnip
Comfrey

EXFOLIANTS
Catsfoot
Complexion brush
Cuckoopint
Lemon Juice
Loofah
Papaya
Pineapple
Tomato

FEET
Agrimony
Alder
Burdock
Goats Rue
Lavender
Massage
Mustard Seed
Pine Needles
Red Clover
Sage
Witch Hazel
Wormwood in Rum

FINGERNAILS
Almond Meal

Honey
Kid Gloves
Dulse
Gelatin
Honey
Kelp
Lanolin
Protein
Silicon
Wheat Germ Oil to
    Massage Cuticle

HAIR, Conditioner
Basil Oil
Cherry Bark
Lavender Oil
Nettle and
    Cherry Bark
Ragwort
Rosemary

HAIR, Dandruff
(see Dandruff)

HAIR, Dark
Apple Cider Vinegar
Bergamot
Clove
Creosote
Henna
Jaborandi
Nettle
Raspberry
Rosemary
Sage
Southernwood

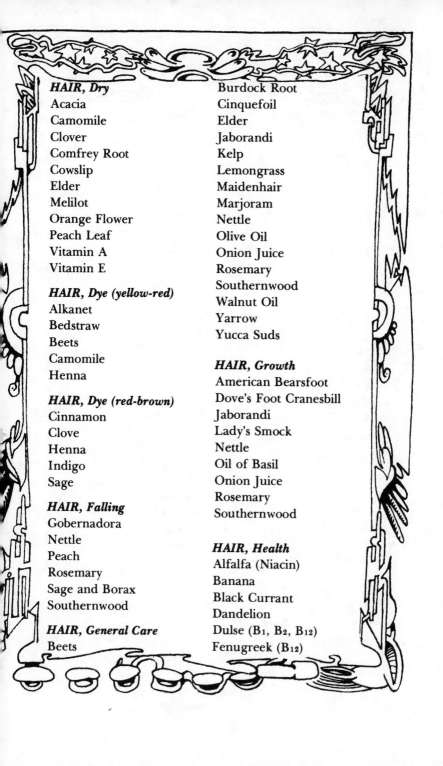

HAIR, Dry
Acacia
Camomile
Clover
Comfrey Root
Cowslip
Elder
Melilot
Orange Flower
Peach Leaf
Vitamin A
Vitamin E

HAIR, Dye (yellow-red)
Alkanet
Bedstraw
Beets
Camomile
Henna

HAIR, Dye (red-brown)
Cinnamon
Clove
Henna
Indigo
Sage

HAIR, Falling
Gobernadora
Nettle
Peach
Rosemary
Sage and Borax
Southernwood

HAIR, General Care
Beets

Burdock Root
Cinquefoil
Elder
Jaborandi
Kelp
Lemongrass
Maidenhair
Marjoram
Nettle
Olive Oil
Onion Juice
Rosemary
Southernwood
Walnut Oil
Yarrow
Yucca Suds

HAIR, Growth
American Bearsfoot
Dove's Foot Cranesbill
Jaborandi
Lady's Smock
Nettle
Oil of Basil
Onion Juice
Rosemary
Southernwood

HAIR, Health
Alfalfa (Niacin)
Banana
Black Currant
Dandelion
Dulse (B_1, B_2, B_{12})
Fenugreek (B_{12})

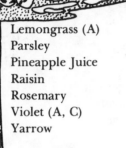

Lemongrass (A)
Parsley
Pineapple Juice
Raisin
Rosemary
Violet (A, C)
Yarrow

HAIR, Light
Camomile
Comfrey Root
Cowslip Flower
Elder Flower
Grapefruit Peel
Lemon Peel
Marigold
Mullein, Yellow
Orange Peel
Orris Root
Quassia
White Willow Bark

HAIR, Oily
Bergamot
Lemongrass
Lemon Peel
Orris Root
Peppermint Oil
Quassia Chip
Rosebuds
Strawberry
Vitamins B2, B6
White Willow Bark
Witch Hazel Bark

HAIR, Scalp
Birch
Coltsfoot
Horsetail
Rosemary
Speedwell
Yarrow

HAIR, Shiny
Camomile
Lemon Peel
Maidenhair Fern
Marigold
Nettle
Quassia
Raspberry
Rosemary
Sage

HAIR, Split Ends
Basil Oil
Lavender Oil
Nutmeg Oil
Olive Oil
Origanum Oil
Peanut Oil
Rosemary Oil
Walnut Oil

HANDS
Camomile
Comfrey Root and Leaf
Fennel
Lady's Mantle

Malva
Marigold
Sage

HEADACHE, Cause
Alcohol
Chocolate

HEADACHE, Cure
Fructose
Honey
Ripe Fruit
Rose Oil
Tomato Juice
Vegetable Juice
Violet Oil

HERPES
Lemon Juice
Walnut Bark
White Willow Bark
Yogurt

HIPS
Dittany
Strawberry Leaf

HYDRATE
Camomile
Honey
Orange Blossoms
Rosebuds
White Willow Bark

HYPNOTIC
Orange Flowers

INFLAMMATION
Comfrey Root
Houseleek
Marshmallow Root
Sandalwood

ITCHES
Agrimony
Aloe
Celandine
Dandelion
Fuchsia
Golden Seal
Parsley
Rosemary
Sage

KNEES
Comfrey
Thyme

LEGS
Dittany of Crete
Hyssop
Iris
Marigold
Pine Needles
Sage
White Pond Lily Root

MUSCLES
Camomile
Comfrey Root
Lavender

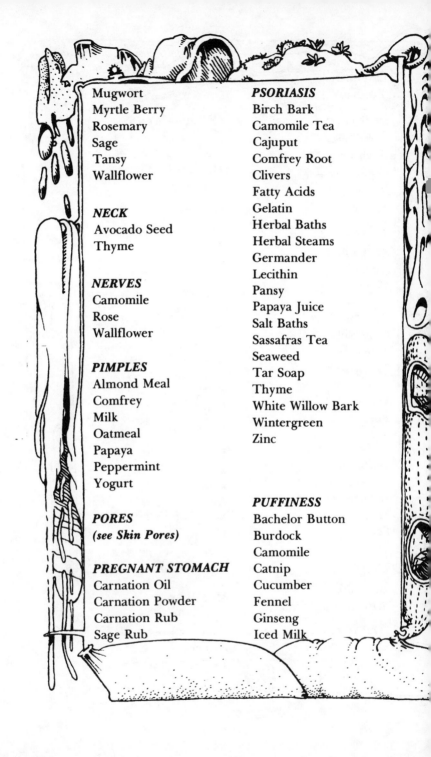

Mugwort
Myrtle Berry
Rosemary
Sage
Tansy
Wallflower

NECK
Avocado Seed
Thyme

NERVES
Camomile
Rose
Wallflower

PIMPLES
Almond Meal
Comfrey
Milk
Oatmeal
Papaya
Peppermint
Yogurt

PORES
(see Skin Pores)

PREGNANT STOMACH
Carnation Oil
Carnation Powder
Carnation Rub
Sage Rub

PSORIASIS
Birch Bark
Camomile Tea
Cajuput
Comfrey Root
Clivers
Fatty Acids
Gelatin
Herbal Baths
Herbal Steams
Germander
Lecithin
Pansy
Papaya Juice
Salt Baths
Sassafras Tea
Seaweed
Tar Soap
Thyme
White Willow Bark
Wintergreen
Zinc

PUFFINESS
Bachelor Button
Burdock
Camomile
Catnip
Cucumber
Fennel
Ginseng
Iced Milk

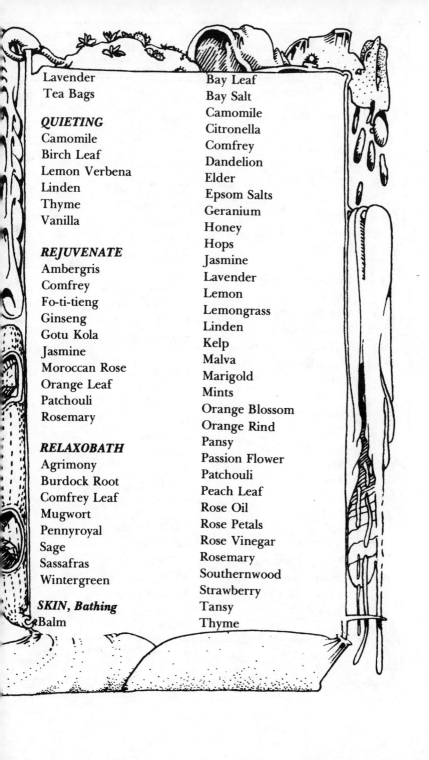

Lavender
Tea Bags

QUIETING
Camomile
Birch Leaf
Lemon Verbena
Linden
Thyme
Vanilla

REJUVENATE
Ambergris
Comfrey
Fo-ti-tieng
Ginseng
Gotu Kola
Jasmine
Moroccan Rose
Orange Leaf
Patchouli
Rosemary

RELAXOBATH
Agrimony
Burdock Root
Comfrey Leaf
Mugwort
Pennyroyal
Sage
Sassafras
Wintergreen

SKIN, Bathing
Balm

Bay Leaf
Bay Salt
Camomile
Citronella
Comfrey
Dandelion
Elder
Epsom Salts
Geranium
Honey
Hops
Jasmine
Lavender
Lemon
Lemongrass
Linden
Kelp
Malva
Marigold
Mints
Orange Blossom
Orange Rind
Pansy
Passion Flower
Patchouli
Peach Leaf
Rose Oil
Rose Petals
Rose Vinegar
Rosemary
Southernwood
Strawberry
Tansy
Thyme

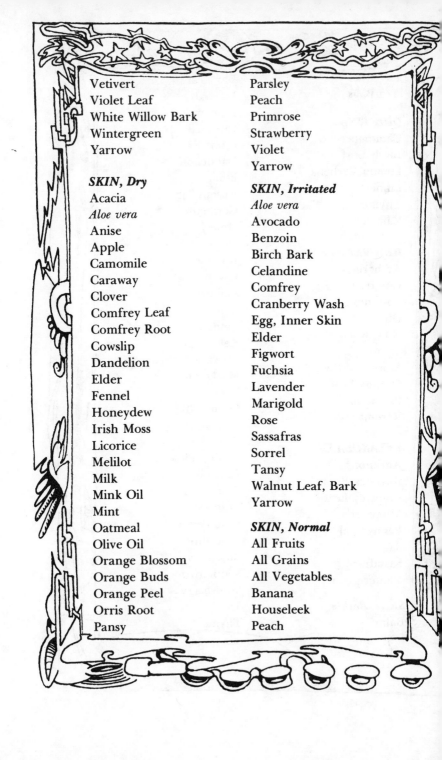

Vetivert
Violet Leaf
White Willow Bark
Wintergreen
Yarrow

SKIN, Dry
Acacia
Aloe vera
Anise
Apple
Camomile
Caraway
Clover
Comfrey Leaf
Comfrey Root
Cowslip
Dandelion
Elder
Fennel
Honeydew
Irish Moss
Licorice
Melilot
Milk
Mink Oil
Mint
Oatmeal
Olive Oil
Orange Blossom
Orange Buds
Orange Peel
Orris Root
Pansy

Parsley
Peach
Primrose
Strawberry
Violet
Yarrow

SKIN, Irritated
Aloe vera
Avocado
Benzoin
Birch Bark
Celandine
Comfrey
Cranberry Wash
Egg, Inner Skin
Elder
Figwort
Fuchsia
Lavender
Marigold
Rose
Sassafras
Sorrel
Tansy
Walnut Leaf, Bark
Yarrow

SKIN, Normal
All Fruits
All Grains
All Vegetables
Banana
Houseleek
Peach

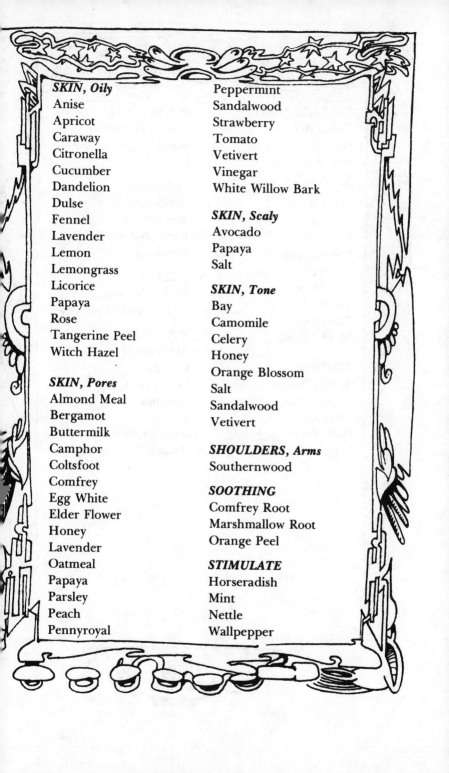

SKIN, Oily
Anise
Apricot
Caraway
Citronella
Cucumber
Dandelion
Dulse
Fennel
Lavender
Lemon
Lemongrass
Licorice
Papaya
Rose
Tangerine Peel
Witch Hazel

SKIN, Pores
Almond Meal
Bergamot
Buttermilk
Camphor
Coltsfoot
Comfrey
Egg White
Elder Flower
Honey
Lavender
Oatmeal
Papaya
Parsley
Peach
Pennyroyal

Peppermint
Sandalwood
Strawberry
Tomato
Vetivert
Vinegar
White Willow Bark

SKIN, Scaly
Avocado
Papaya
Salt

SKIN, Tone
Bay
Camomile
Celery
Honey
Orange Blossom
Salt
Sandalwood
Vetivert

SHOULDERS, Arms
Southernwood

SOOTHING
Comfrey Root
Marshmallow Root
Orange Peel

STIMULATE
Horseradish
Mint
Nettle
Wallpepper

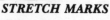

STRETCH MARKS
Cocoa Butter
Carnation Massage
Sage Rub
Vitamin E

SUNBURN
Aloe vera
Comfrey
Lemon Juice
Lettuce
Rice Water
Seaweed
Tea Bags
Witch Hazel

TEETH
Alfalfa Sprouts
Apples, Raw
Clove Oil
Orris Root
Peppermint Oil

Peruvian Bark
Rosemary Powder
Salt
Soda

THROAT
Artichoke
Avocado
Cocoa Butter
Lanolin

TISSUES
Aroma Massage
Camomile, to Strengthen

WRINKLES
Almond Oil
Cowslip
Cuckoopint
Cucumber
Lanolin
Mink Oil
Vitamin E

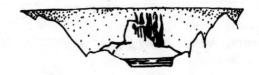

Chapter II

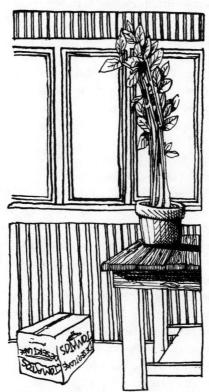

A Cosmetic Glossary
of Useful Terms

Absorbent. A substance that can absorb another, such as a sponge or absorbent cotton.

Acetum. A vinegar solution containing aromatics.

Alterative. A vague term used in herbalism that means a substance that has the ability to slowly change an unhealthy condition to a healthy one.

Anesthetic. A substance that produces loss of sensation.

Anodyne. A painkiller.

Antihydrotic. A substance that reduces the amount of sweat from the sweat glands.

Antipyretic. A substance that reduces fever.

Antiseptic. A substance that inhibits the growth of microorganisms on living tissue.

Aromatherapy. A way of treating mental and physical illness through the inhalation of volatile oils; combining the use of pure essential oils and pressure point therapy to treat illness.

Aromatic. A fragrant-smelling plant or medicine, sometimes with a pleasant taste, sometimes with a strong bitter taste, that is used often to cover the taste of unpleasant drugs or medicines.

Aromatic Water. A clear solution of distilled water saturated with an aromatic such as Orange flower water, Rosewater, Lavender water, or Elder flower water.

Aromemories. Memories associated with various scents.

Astringent. Used in cosmetics for cleaning the skin and/or contracting the pores.

Bactericide. A substance that destroys bacteria.

Bain-Marie. A type of water bath in which fine cosmetics may be prepared (see Water Bath).

Balsam. A substance, usually found in ointments, that soothes and heals. Balsam is the resin that exudes from certain trees and plants.

Bruise. To bruise a leaf or plant to extract its properties is to mash, crush, pulverize, or crunch up that leaf or plant with your fingers, a pestle, or some other implement such as the back of a wooden spoon.

Castile. A hard white soap made originally from the Olive oil of Castile and now generally Olive oil and Tallow; however, the term has been bastardized by the soap companies to mean just about any soap with a concentration of twenty per cent and above Olive oil. Real castile soap would have an Olive oil percentage of forty to fifty per cent and above.

Cerate. A substance made of fats and oils with beeswax added to harden it. Cerates are used externally. An herbal cerate is made with one to four ounces of a mixture of herbs that have been simmered in one pound or more of fats or oils for twenty minutes or so. Some cerates have one ounce of white wine added to keep the oil or fat from having a burned smell. Cool and strain the mixture and add one-half ounce of melted beeswax to every one cup of strained oil and then beat until cold.

Counter-irritant. A substance used to produce a superficial inflammation of the skin to relieve a deeper inflammation of the body. Cayenne pepper is such a substance; i.e., when it is made into a cerate, mellita, or decoction for stimulating hair growth if clogged hair follicles are present.

Decoction. A liquid extract of the hard parts of plants such as the bark, root, or seeds. One to four ounces of the herbs are added to twenty ounces of liquid such as milk, vinegar or water and then boiled or simmered for five to twenty minutes or more. The liquid is strained and the resultant decoction is used for cosmetic or medicinal purposes. Makes about sixteen ounces.

Demulcent. A soothing substance used internally. An infusion or decoction used internally to soothe and protect inflamed mucous surfaces; i.e., Comfrey root decoction for stomach ulcers.

Deodorant. A substance used to cover or inhibit nasty body odors.

Diaphoretic. A substance that makes you perspire.

Disinfectant. A substance that destroys microorganisms that cause disease and create infection.

Diuretic. A substance that causes more free flow and volume from the kidneys flushing the excretory system. Causes more and freer urination.

Elixir. An alcoholic substance—about twenty-five per cent alcohol—sweetened, used for medicinal purpose.

One method of making an elixir is to take one ounce mixed herbs and add eight ounces boiling water. Simmer for about ten minutes, using a nonmetal pot with top. Take off heat, add sugar to taste and steep until cold, then strain. Add about eight ounces of 100-proof vodka. Set aside for use. Depending on the ailment, take a teaspoon or so every hour or, for a child, every four hours. (See also Syrup.)

Enfleurage. The cold extraction of the volatile flower oil by using fat on frames or plates for absorption.

Emollient. An infusion or decoction used externally to soothe and protect inflamed mucous surfaces; i.e., Comfrey root decoction for pain of arthritis. Any soothing protecting substance used externally such as lanolin hand cream.

Emulsion. A substance made up of totally different components which, when combined, stay combined such as the egg, oil, and vinegar ingredients in cosmetic mayonnaise.

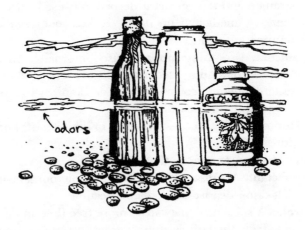

Essence. One ounce pure essential oil of herb dissolved in one or two cups of alcohol or two cups 100-proof vodka, or ¼ ounce oil to 4 ounces 50 per cent alcohol.

Essential Oil. That part of the plant that possesses the fragrance of the plant or flower in concentrated form. Essential oil is usually obtained by steam distillation while extraction by fats (enfleurage) is usually called a flower oil.

Eye Cream. A cream made up especially for the delicate thin oil-poor skin around the eyes, and made of a finer texture for better penetration. The best eye cream is pure vitamin E applied directly from a capsule.

Exfoliant. A substance used in either lotion, cream, or mask form, which contains a mild peeling agent to help clear the skin of its residue of dead skin cells, which sometimes accumulate and make the skin dull and sallow.

Extract. A concentrated product made by treating a natural raw material with a solvent.

Exudate. That which oozes from a wound or sore of a plant, person, or other animal.

Firming Cream. A cream said to improve the superficial appearance of the skin by tightening the skin surface.

Fixative. A substance that "fixes" or sets the volatile ingredients in another substance from evaporating too quickly.

Fomentation. Applying heat and moisture through the use of wet cloths to reduce an inflammation or ease pain. A poultice.

Herb. In Webster's unabridged dictionary the word is defined as: 1. A seed-producing annual, biannual, or herbaceous perennial that does not develop persistent woody tissue but dies down at the end of a growing season—compared to shrub or tree (a definition for botanists). 2. A plant *or* plant part valued for its medicinal, savory, or aromatic qualities (a definition for the old herbalists as well as modern herbalists which includes any part of shrubs, trees, flowers, etc., any living plant). 3. The leafy top of an herbaceous plant considered separately from its root (this definition is used in herbal cosmetic recipes).

Herbal. A book in which plants are described and named and their uses defined.

Herbalism. The oldest healing art in the world; the art of healing by the use of nonpoisonous herbs, administered externally or internally, usually using the whole plant without eliminating any part.

Herbalist. One who grows, collects, studies, and uses plants medicinally or cosmetically. My daughter defines an herbalist as "someone who makes cosmetics and stuff like shampoos out of green things that look like weeds." An herbalist also practices the art of healing by using plants; also called an herb doctor.

Herbologist. One who studies the uses of plants and may also grow, collect, and discourse about them.

Herbology. The science of studying the uses of plants for cosmetic and especially medicinal purposes.

Homeopathy. A system of healing using very small doses of a plant or drug material. In healthy persons this would produce the symptoms of the disease being treated; i.e., using onion for a person with a cold who has a runny nose and eyes; if used on a healthy person he would get a runny nose and eyes.

Hormone Cream. A firming cream containing synthetic estrogens that only temporarily firms, smooths, and plumps up skin. Should only be used upon advice from a dermatologist.

Humectant. Something which helps the skin retain moisture, usually a liquid.

Hydrating. The ability to restore or maintain the normal fluid proportion in the skin or body. Hydrating agents are used in cosmetics to keep the skin natural, moist, firm, and young-looking.

Infusion. The resultant liquid when boiling water is poured onto an herb, the herb infused or soaked for a period of time. Decoctions are simmered or boiled and are usually composed of the hard parts of a plant such as the root, bark, or seed, while the infusion is made chiefly from the softer parts, such as the flower, leaf, or herb. To make an infusion bring twenty ounces water to a boil and pour over one to four ounces herb (using a nonmetal pot), simmer a minute, turn off heat, and steep, or infuse, for five to twenty minutes depending on the use and material involved. Strain and use.

Inhalation. A method of treating mental and physical problems through the inhalation of the volatile oils of medicinal or aromatic plants rather than the drinking or injecting of them.

Irritant. A substance that irritates, such as poison oak or Nettles.

Liquor. A solution of medicinal substances in water as distinguished from a tincture, which is a solution of substances in alcohol.

Lotion. A substance, usually a liquid, that is applied externally to the hands, body, or face for its softening, medicinal, cosmetic, cleansing, or astringent qualities.

Lubrication Cream. A substance, usually semisolid, used to soothe and soften extra dry skin, usually made of oils.

Medicinal. A remedy or substance used in treating physical or mental disease.

Mellita. An infusion or decoction mixed or made with honey, instead of sugar, to sweeten it. One method is to make an infusion or decoction, strain it, and to eight ounces add four ounces or more of honey.

Moisturizer. Something which helps the skin retain its natural moisture or adds moisture and is usually a liquid or a lotion. (See Humectant.)

Mucilage. A substance that swells up in water without dissolving and forms a slimy, sticky, or gelatinous mass. The mucilage is used as an adhesive in incense, a demulcent in medicine, or an emollient in cosmetics. To make a mucilage with Irish Moss, simmer one ounce of the seaweed with one quart of liquid for some time, at least until the weed is very gooey and has absorbed much of the liquid. Strain through cheese-cloth into a bowl and wring cloth until quite dry. To make a mucilage with Gum Tragacanth . . . "take a teaspoon of powdered Tragacanth and add water, a bit at a time, until it becomes a nice sticky gooey mess about the consistency of uncooked egg white." (*Herbs & Things*, p. 250.)

Nervine. An agent that soothes the nerves.

Night Cream. A cream usually used on the face at night, for moisturizing, stopping surface evaporation, or plumping up the skin to get rid of lines and wrinkles.

Oxymel. Made from water, honey and vinegar in the proportion of five parts honey to one part water to one part vinegar.

Pharmacognosy. The science encompassing those phases of knowledge relating to natural products which are generally of medicinal value and primarily of plant origin.

Pledget. A bit of cotton or other substance used to apply medication, cosmetics, or aromatics or to absorb another substance.

Poultice. A heated soft mass of macerated, bruised fresh herbs spread on cloth and applied directly to the aching or bruised area to cause increased circulation and sweating and to get rid of impurities when used as a facial. A hot cloth is applied over the herbal mass to keep it hot. An herb or fruit applied directly without heat can also be a poultice; e.g., pear.

Restorative. An agent used to bring a person or a part of that person back to normal vigor.

Rubefacient. An external agent used to cause redness of the skin.

Salve. A soothing or healing medicinal or cosmetic ointment.

Sedative. A substance which has a soothing or calming effect.

Spirit. An essence or a ten per cent alcohol solution, a liquid produced by distillation. A simple spirit is one composed of one ounce herb to six ounces 100-proof vodka, soaked, macerated, shaken, and steeped for two weeks, and then strained and about twelve ounces of water added.

Stimulant. A substance that only temporarily quickens the activity or the tissues; e.g., massage.

Styptic. A substance that contracts the tissues, such as Alum on a cold sore.

Synergist. A substance which when combined with another increases the effectiveness of both.

Syrup. An infusion or decoction made with sugar to sweeten it. Make an infusion or decoction, cool it, strain it and to every four ounces add about one ounce or more of sugar. Bottle and refrigerate.

Tea. An infusion used cosmetically, medicinally, or as a beverage. Bring ten ounces water to a boil in a covered nonmetal pot and pour it over one teaspoon to one

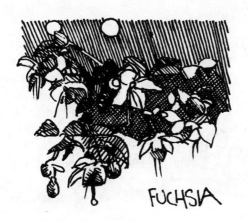

FUCHSIA

tablespoon herb (depending on the strength you like) in a preheated pot. Turn off the heat and steep one to five minutes, strain, and use.

Throat Cream. A cream used for the throat that has a rich or thick texture and is used to help keep the neck area (low in oil glands and thin-skinned) moisturized to prevent lines from forming.

Tincture. An alcoholic solution containing medicinals or aromatics, about fifty per cent alcohol. To make, infuse one to four ounces herbs directly into one cup of 100-proof alcohol such as vodka, shake daily for ten days, strain, and use.

Tisane. A nourishing decoction, often having a slight medicinal quality, originally one made from Barley. Now it is often used for a beverage tea made from flowers. (Also can be defined as an infusion of herbs.)

Tonic. A substance, usually a liquid, that invigorates, restores, or stimulates the system to improve health or body tone.

Unguent. A preparation made from fat or oil usually for medicinal or cosmetic purpose that liquefies upon application to the body.

Venetian. Olive oil soap usually containing a higher percentage of Olive oil than castile soap.

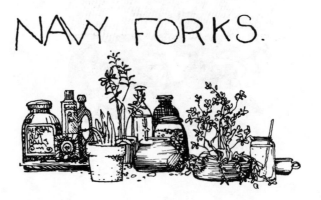

Water Bath. Also known as a *bain-marie*. A pot containing water in which is placed another pot containing the substance being cooked; used for cooking delicate or sensitive ingredients.

For further definitions of herbal terms see *Herbs & Things*. Jeanne Rose's Herbal, which furnished a few of the above definitions.

Chapter III

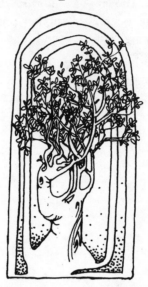

Descriptions of Many of the Plants (and Other Things) Useful on the Body

. . . By following nature, we cannot fail.
—*Michel de Montaigne*

THE SUBSTANCES MARKED 🔥 HAVE BEEN KNOWN
TO HAVE CAUSED IRRITATION, ALLERGIC REACTIONS,
OR SENSITIVITIES ON SOME PEOPLE. HOWEVER, ALL
SUBSTANCES HAVE BEEN IMPLICATED TO SOME DEGREE
IN UNPLEASANT REACTIONS ON SOMEONE, SO IT WOULD
BE WISE TO TRY THE PATCH TEST BEFORE USING A NEW
PLANT OR OTHER COSMETIC SUBSTANCE EXTERNALLY.

THE PATCH TEST. If you have sensitive skin or a history of allergies, then by all means use a patch test to test your relative sensitivity to the new ingredients. To try out a new, store-bought cosmetic, a homemade cosmetic, or any new plant that you are unfamiliar with when making your own cosmetics, make a paste of the plant with water and apply to your forearm in an area about the size of a quarter. Let the paste dry there and apply a loose Band-Aid. If there is no reaction within twenty-four hours—terrific—go ahead and use the plant or cosmetic. Apply creams or lotions to the forearm directly, apply Band-Aid for twenty-four hours, and check arm for reaction. By all means, keep all alien substances away from the eyes.

HERBS are annotated in the text by various initials or words as follows:

Po—powdered—When an herb has been finely powdered.
Gr—ground—More coarsely powdered than a powder.
Cs—cut and sifted—The plant material is dried and then coarsely cut up, and any extraneous material or powder sifted out.
Pc—pieces—Usually large pieces of bark.
Wh—whole—You will usually want to purchase your flowers and seeds whole rather than in any other form. Seeds, of course, will be more potent if you grind them yourself, and of course, flowers are prettier when used whole.

🜚 **Acacia, Gum** (*Acacia senegal*) Also called Gum Arabic. This gum is slowly soluble in water and provides a gelatinous acid base for nonoily cosmetics. It makes a demulcent and emollient base, very soothing to all skin surfaces.

🜚 **Acacia flowers** (*Acacia sp.*) Otherwise known as Sweet Acacia. The Cassie (*Acacia farnesiana*) and the Mimosa, (*A. decurrens dealbata*) are members of this group and are used cosmetically in the same way. Fresh, these flowers are extracted or macerated in order to extract the essential oil which is usually so expensive that most of us will only be able to afford the poor synthetic. They are grown all over the world but most perfumers use the flowers grown in southern France, Syria, or Provence. Dried, they are used in bath herbs especially for dry skins, in facial steamers

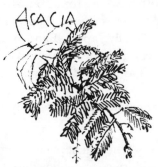

to improve the complexion, in potpourris for a violet or floral note. The Acacia tree in my backyard produces the most gorgeous bright yellow blossoms in the spring (February and March) which, in San Francisco, is especially nice. And the scent that wafts about the yard is divine, although some of my friends claim that it makes them sneeze. I pay my little girl to pick the blossoms, and it is a delight to see her climb to the very top of the tree with just her head peeking out between the yellow balls of fluff. And then, of course, for weeks afterwards we make yummy, smelly, yellow potpourris and take baths with pounds of Acacia flowers. Our skin smells good and feels so silky.

Agrimony (*Agrimonia eupatoria*) is used in herbal baths to help sore muscles feel better, and as an external application (decoction form) for pimples and skin eruptions.

Alder (*Alder sp.*) Black, tag, and common Alder barks,

when soaked in vinegar and mixed with other cleansing herbs, are useful as a wash for skin irritations and also as an ingredient in herbal baths for swellings, inflammations and rheumatism-type complaints. Black Alder taken internally as a tea is said to be useful for skin problems.

🔥**Alfalfa** (*Medicago sativa*) Even the poor Alfalfa, which is so nourishing when eaten, has caused irritations and allergic reactions on some sensitive skins. But most of us can use this wonderful plant, which occasionally grows roots up to 128 feet long, in facial steams as a very mild exfoliant (it contains protease, a protein digester); in creams and oils, as herbal bath mixtures for its healing qualities and chlorophyll content; and in protein hair rinses. Try a gritty mixture of Alfalfa-Gr and Papaya pulp as a facial mask.

Alkanet (*Alkanna tinctoria, Lithosperum tinctorium*) A nonirritating red dye plant whose color can be controlled and is used in the making of lipstick, face glazers, and with Henna as a nail color. A wine decoction of Alkanet is used as a rub for sore backs. An ointment of Alkanet is sometimes used for sores, bruises, and cuts.

🔥**Allspice** (*Pimenta officinalis*) Used in hair rinses for its brown color and nice spicy scent; in perfume and cologne; astringent and freshener making; and in bath herbs, ointments, and creams for its slight anesthetic effect. Generally it is used in powdered rather than cut form.

Almond meal (Sweet Almond—*Amygdalus communis,* var. *dulcis, Prunis communis,* var. *dulcis*) Sweet Almonds, when ripe and shelled, are ground up into a meal and used as beauty grains for the slight bleaching action on the skin; in scrubs for their cleansing and emollient quality; and mixed into soaps for the scrubbing effect and bleaching quality. Almond milk is used in lotions.

Almond, oil of Sweet (*Prunis communis dulcis*) is identical with the other fruit kernel oils, such as Apricot and Peach. It is used in the same way and can be substituted for these other oils, which are nondrying and therefore very useful on dry skin. These oils are also used in all sorts of fine cosmetics for their excellent emolliency. They can also be used in cooking.

☾ **Almond, oil of Bitter** (*Prunis amygdalus,* var. *amara*) is an essential oil used to scent fine cosmetics and in the making of heliotrope and muguet perfumes. It is also used to scent soaps. Everyone (at least almost everyone) likes the scent of the Bitter Almond but there are many who develop sensitivity to this oil, especially when it is used in soaps. It is also used to scent "violet" potpourris. Bitter Almond kernels, as well as Peach kernels, Apricot kernels, and Apple seeds, contain glucose, prussic (hydrocyanic) acid, and the essential oil, benzaldehyde. People who eat fresh Apricot or Peach kernels for their health should be made aware of this fact as they are endangering their very life if they happen to eat too many kernels. Of course you can develop a tolerance for cyanide poisoning by eating a few kernels at a time and slowly increasing the daily dose. An acquaintance of mine tells a story about a friend of his who loved fresh Apple seeds from the time he was a child until he died. He loved them so much that finally he started saving them up from every Apple he and his family ate until soon he had about a cupful of Apple seeds. He sat down and ate every one of them and died within the day of cyanide poisoning. It is a law that when you buy an essential oil containing prussic acid as one of its constituents, the prussic acid has to be removed. The label will usually read: Bitter Almond, FFPA (meaning Free from Prussic Acid), or Bitter Almond, NF (meaning National Formulary, which is just about the same thing as FFPA).

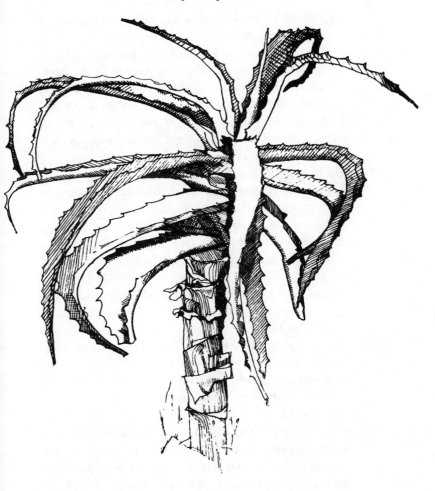

Aloe The Aloe usually referred to is the *Aloe vera,*
although it is also known as *A. barbadensis,* and lives
normally in the Canary Islands. The Aloe here in San
Francisco often confused with *vera* is *A. arborescens*
(tree-like aloe). *Vera* is an indispensable plant for the
homemaker. It is incredibly useful for any type of
burn you may get and when it grows large and juicy, it's
super in all sorts of creams, lotions, shampoos, and on

all parts of the body for cuts, scratches, bruises, sore or irritated skin, for burns, sunburns, X-ray burns, bug bites, and any other skin problems you can imagine. *Aloe vera* grows anywhere in my house: in the bathroom, where there is no sun; on top of the display case, where it gets no water; on the living room table, where there is sun and, at night, fog and wind; on the oven, where it is usually warm; and outside, where it gets red and windblown. The only thing it does not like is the cold, in which it dies. But how do you tell the various Aloes apart? *Aloe vera* grows thick juicy leaves only minimally thorny while the *A. arborescens* with which it is confused has a stalk-like base and thinner, thornier leaves. However, we have found that once when we took an *arborescens* on a desert trip instead of a *vera* it performed just as well in the healing department. To use the plant for a small cut or burn, cut off a small, say one-half-inch section, and slit it lengthwise to expose the gelatinous part; apply this to the wound or sunburn. While on a vacation with friends and toasting at the beach in Santa Cruz, Joanna's young baby was left much too long in the sun and received a very severe striped sunburn (he was under a slatted canvas chair). When we brought him in he was screeching with pain but fortunately we had a *vera* growing outside the house. I cut a two-foot section of the leaf blade, split it lengthwise, applied the gooey side to the baby's back and left it there about five minutes. He went to sleep right away, and when he woke up his slatted sunburn had turned into a striped tan. For creams, lotions, or hair treatments add about one ounce of the clear gelatinous matter—obtained from the leaf of the plant by scraping or cutting it out—to about three ounces of the cream, lotion, or shampoo; mix thoroughly or blend in the blender. For homemade soap, check the soap chapter for how to use the *vera*.

🌿 **Alum root** (*Geranium maculatum, Heuchera americana*) The root of the Geranium is extremely astringent and is used externally to dry up sores, as an ingredient in herbal douches, as a deodorizing wash, and in herbal baths for oily skin.

🌿 **Amaranth** (*Amaranthus hypochondriacus*) If you can get the fresh Amaranth, use it in cosmetics for its healing qualities or in herbal baths mixed with other scented plants. It is slightly astringent and good in wrinkle creams with added vitamin E.

Ambergris or whale exudate from *Physeter catodon* is used as a fine (and rather expensive) fixative in perfumes and potpourris and is added to cosmetics for its light pleasant scent. It is used in the form of an extract made by macerating the raw stuff in alcohol. Tincture of Ambergris is available at Caswell-Massey, that venerable old New York pharmacy.

Ambrette seed (*Hibiscus abelmoschus, H. moscheutes*) A seed from a type of Hibiscus which has a musky odor and is used in musk perfumes as a fixative. It is also used in potpourris and in cosmetics for this same musky odor.

🌿 **Anemone** (*Anemone pulsatilla*) The Anemones—wind flowers or pasque flowers—are used in their entirety for various cutaneous problems including plant rashes. And for some reason, they are especially recommended for fair, blue-eyed women.

Anise (*Pimpinella anisum;* the star Anise is *Illicium verum, I. anisatum*) The seed of the Anise smells somewhat like Licorice and is mixed with spirits of wine to make the liqueur, anisette. It is used cosmetically in facial steams to open and medicate the pores. It is also very useful in hair rinses for its color, cleansing action on the scalp pores, and wonderful scent.

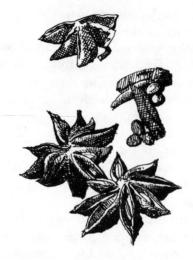

☙ **Annatto** (*Bixa orellana*) The dried pulp of the fruit of this
plant is available in herb stores and is used as coloring
matter in lipstick, face glazers, rouge, and hair rinses.

Apple (*Pyrus malus*) Apple cider is especially nice diluted
with a bit of water as a natural astringent and can be
used "straight" as a hair setting lotion. Apple pips
contain prussic acid and are dangerous (see Almond,
oil of bitter). Mashed fresh pulp of Apple is slightly
acid and is used in all sorts of masks, hand creams, and
scrubs for roughness of skin; it is especially effective
on sensitive or fair skins. An excellent pomade for
rough skin, elbows, heels, and knees is made by mixing Apple pulp with equal amounts of solid fat and
rosewater; the ingredients can be altered to suit your
needs. Apple pulp and honey is terrific for soothing
dry, irritated, or sensitive skin.

Apricot (*Prunus armeniaca*) Apricot pulp is terrific for
those with a tendency to sallow or oily skin. You can
use fresh, dried and soaked, or powdered Apricot
mixed with just about anything you can think of such
as milk, sour cream, yogurt, water, or Apricot wine, as

a scrub or mask, to help those enlarged or oily pores. Apricot kernel oil is used in creams and lotions, salves and pomades. The oil and pulp are useful in all sorts of cosmetics, soaps, and cold creams. A synthetic substance called Apricot "essence" is available if you care to use it.

🕯 **Arnica** (*Arnica Montana*) The flowers are used in an infusion for the feet to strengthen and toughen them or to help cure athlete's foot. Arnica can also be used as a hair rinse with Jaborandi or Nettle to stimulate growth. A thick decoction of the flowers is used as a daily scalp massage lotion for growth but this can occasionally produce inflammation when overused.

🕯 **Arrowroot** (*Maranta arundinacea, Canna edulis, Curcuma augustifolia*) The tuberous rhizomes of several plants yield the starch called Arrowroot. It is sometimes used mixed with water and applied as a paste to the body or face to help dry up pimples or for other sores or wounds.

Artichoke (*Cynara scolymus*) The globe Artichoke leaves are used as an excellent detergent rinse for dandruff and make a very useful addition to a dandruff rinse especially when mixed with Comfrey and Willow bark. You can use either the leaves from the plant proper or the leaves from the globe after you have eaten the good part. You can also use the water, in which you have cooked the Artichokes, straight. I have a letter from Sibyl who received a letter from Crystal who lives in Saigon that states, ". . . Artichoke leaves are a LIVER ELIXIR. . . . Crystal had a horrible skin flare-up and her Vietnamese maid made her a tea every day of Artichoke leaves; apparently the tea cleared up her skin problem right away"—the tea was drunk every day and also applied as an external wash.

🕯 **Asclepias** There are many species of this plant, and most, when used in the bath, act as a mild diaphoretic and are therefore effective in opening the pores and getting rid of impurities. The fresh flowers of *A. syriaca,* a Milkweed, have dull red-to-purply fragrant flowers, which are welcome additions to the bath. And along with the young shoots, these flowers can also be eaten. Gibbons tells how to cook them in his book, *Stalking the Wild Asparagus,* p. 132. The seeds of some species are silky and are combined with other herbs in my Sleep Pillows. Milkweed juice, which is milky, is used daily as an external application to get rid of warts and pimples. And some of the Milkweeds have very potent insecticidal properties and can be used dried and spread around the room and under rugs to get rid of fleas. Fifty years ago there were many brands of Milkweed cream (for the face and body); one, that I have, promises to "keep the skin soft, smooth, and velvety, is delightful to use, prevents chapping and roughness and is readily absorbed and is used for tan, freckles, and sunburn." It also contains a cautionary note that "when the system is in a bad condition a too liberal use of Milkweed Cream may, by overstimulating the skin, temporarily exaggerate its defects. It should then be used more sparingly—but persistently, and more often."

Ash (*Fraxinus excelsior,* European Ash; *F. spp.,* Common or Weeping Ash) Grieve, *A Modern Herbal,* says the Ash had the reputation of magically curing warts; each wart must be pricked with a new pin that has been thrust into the tree, the pins are withdrawn and left in the tree, and the following charm is repeated:

> *Ashen tree, ashen tree,*
> *Pray buy these warts of me.*

Asparagus (*Asparagus officinalis*) spears are used in many stimulating facial washes to cleanse the face and act to dry up pimples and sores. Mixed with yogurt they make an excellent facial mask.

AVOCADOS

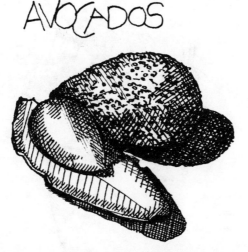

Avocado (*Persea americana*) The Alligator Pear contains
vitamins A, D, E, and potassium, sulfur, and chlorine.
Avocados are used in facial and scalp packs for their
penetrating power. The oil is used in combination
with other less penetrating but also less drying oils as a
conveyor of these vitamins to the skin and the glands
of the skin. The meat, seed, peel, and oil all have their
special place in cosmetic preparations. *The Fresh Avocado Beauty Book* is completely devoted to the myriad
uses of the Avocado. I especially like to eat big fat
home-grown Florida Avocados baked and stuffed
with chicken or the rough-skinned Avocado with Garlic in blue corn tortillas.

Balm (*Melissa offinalis*) also called Sweet Balm, Lemon
Balm, or Melissa. It smells wonderfully lemony, is
delicious as a tea mixed with Rosemary to help the
memory and for melancholy, and is best used fresh
rather than dried. It is also used with Jaborandi and
Nettle for hair growth, as a rinse or in shampoos, and
mixed with other lemon-scented plants (Lemon,
Lemongrass) in facial steams to correct skin
blemishes.

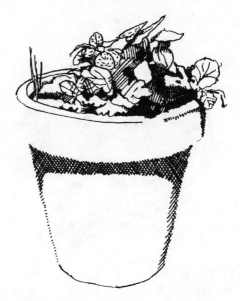

Balm of Gilead buds (*Populus candicans, Commiphora opobalsamum;* no relation to the Balm of Gilead fir, *Abies balsamea*) are used by mashing and simmering in oil and applying this oil externally for skin diseases. When mixed with Jamaican rum and steeped for a few days, the resultant liquor can be drunk for coughs and colds or applied locally for sores, bruises, and cuts. Freshly dried buds, if you can get them, are wonder-

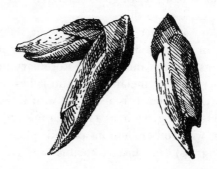

fully aromatic and rather stickily moist and can be squeezed open, the resin being used as an unguent or dotted onto pimples to heal them. The buds look rather like the brown mummified chrysalis of an exotic butterfly.

Balsam of Peru (*Myroxylon balsamum,* var. *pereirae* and other varieties) is used straight as a disinfectant for various types of skin disease including eczema, pruritis, and prurigo; to relieve the itch of scabies and to kill the eggs; for sores and ringworm; and as an external and toughening application for sore nipples. (It seems to promote healthy epithelial growth and should be mixed with castor oil before adding to your skin ointments.) It is wonderfully and deliciously fragrant and is used in soaps—including medicinal soaps—for chapped hands and feet. The Balsam is soluble in alcohol and is effective as a potent fixative in perfumery and potpourris.

Balsam of Tolu (*Toluifera balsamum, Myroxylon balsamum, Myrosperum toluiferum*) is available from Indiana Botanic and is used much the same as Balsam of Peru, the scent being vanilla-like and somewhat cinnamony. It is employed as a fixative in perfumery or potpourris, in pharmaceutical preparations and soapmaking.

Banana (*Musa paradisiaca, M. spp.*) mashed, makes an excellent, nourishing facial mask for normal to dry skin that can be eaten for its flavorful, tropical deliciousness.

Barberry, European (*Berberis vulgaris*) is used in shampoos and herbal hair rinses. In the *Magic of Herbs,* Mrs. Leyel says, "To cause the hair to grow: 'Take the barberry and fill an iron pot therewith, fill it up with as much water as it will contain, then boil on a slow fire to the half. With this water wash your head morning and evening. Take care that the wash does not touch any part where the hair should not grow.' "

Barley (*Hordeum spp.*) is occasionally used, slightly cooked and mashed with milk, as a cleansing, healing facial mask and toner. Take a Barley water bath for soothing sore, achey flesh.

Basil (*Ocimum minimum*—Bush Basil, *Ocimum basilicum* —Sweet Basil; also spelled *Ocymum*) th`at wonderfully delicious smelling herb which loses most of its olfactory delight upon drying, is best used fresh and is an absolutely imperative ingredient when making turtle soup or pesto sauce. The essential oil of Basil is used as an expensive hair dressing mixed with Lavender oil to perfume the hair and as a tonic to help in hair growth and to reduce tangles and snarls. Rosemary oil is a cheap but effective substitute for the Basil-Lavender mixture. Arabian women are said to powder Basil and Lavender and to brush it into the hair to perfume it.

Bayberry (*Myrica cerifera*) also called Wax Myrtle, is used in the making of candles, soaps, and to scent various cosmetics, especially masculine types. The wax is also employed in the making of aromatic, softening shaving lather. Myrtle wax from the berries is used to make aromatic candles, as an ingredient in soapmaking or shaving soaps, or as an aftershave lotion. The leaves are aromatic and the bark is astringent.

Bay Laurel, The Noble Bay, *Laurus nobilis,* and the California Bay, *Umbellularia Californica,* are potent stimulating antiseptics, used wherever stimulation is needed as in facial or hair packs or in herbal bath mixtures for aching joints and muscles. The scent is inhaled for congested respiration and can be used in aromatherapy. The California Bay, when inhaled a little, will cure a headache but if overused can cause a headache. Bay leaf oil in hair lotions and aftershave is from *Pimenta racemosa.*

Bean flowers, various species of *Phaseolus,* and the water made by distillation, are used in all kinds of lotions and skin tonics. The water is cooling and excellent for a baby's delicate skin. It is used as a wash for all sorts of skin irritations or skin disease including dry scruffy scalps and dandruff. It is also effective in shampoos and hair rinses. The Kidney Bean was an Egyptian object of sacred worship and was venerated for thousands of years.

Bearsfoot (*Polymnia uvedalia*) is said to be used externally in lotions that stimulate hair growth, especially mixed with Southernwood and Jaborandi.

Beech (*Fagus sylvatica*—European white beech) tar is an externally applied antiseptic for skin problems.

Beet (*Beta vulgaris*) juice is especially nice as a face wash or tonic. A bit of mashed, cooked Beets mixed with yogurt makes an excellent facial mask. The juice can be dribbled on talcum or powdered eggshells to color them a soft pink, or in make-up such as rouge and lipstick.

Benzoin gum (*Styrax benzoin*—Sumatra, and *S. tonkinensis*—Siam) is used as an external application for fungus and mold infections of the skin; as an ingredient in various lotions, potions, and cosmetics to retard darkening and to act as a cosmetic preservative. The gum is also used as a fixative in sachets, incense, and potpourris and is a wonderful addition to soaps. The tincture is used also as an external application for the treatment of various skin irritations, mixed with glycerin or lanolin for chapped hands and lips and for irritated overused nipples. It is antiseptic, a mild stimulant, a preservative of fats and is rapidly absorbed.

Bergamot (*Citrus bergamia*) The rind of this nonedible citrus fruit yields an oil by expression that is used in toilet water, cologne, floral and heavy perfumes, and in soaps. The oil is used in inhalation therapy to cause sleep; in suntan preparations, it increases the skin's ability to tan and should therefore not be used on sensitive skin. It has a wonderfully fresh, sweet fragrance and is grown commercially only in Calabria, the southwestern toe of the Italian peninsula. It is often added to greasy hair preparations and sometimes causes skin sensitivities especially on the forehead.

🔥 **Bergamot** is also called Bee Balm, Oswego Tea, or *Monarda didyma* (a substitute is American Horsemint or *M. punctata*), and is used externally in facial masks as a rubefacient, in facial steams, in beverage teas to cleanse the system. The oil is occasionally used to scent soaps and cosmetics.

Bergamot mint See Mint, orange.

🔥 **Betel** (*Piper betel*) leaves are used externally, I am told, as a poultice to relieve skin secretions and are especially useful to suppress mammary secretions. They also act as an antiseptic in various types of abscess.

Betony wood (*Stachys officinalis, S. betonica, Betony officinalis, Betonia officinalis*) also called Bishop's Wort, is used as a compress for headaches and, more often, is taken internally as tea rather than used externally as a cosmetic, although it enjoys a great reputation as a protection against witchcraft.

🔥 **Birch bark** (*Betula alba* and *B. spp.*) is used for its fragrant odor, antiseptic quality, and salicylic acid content. A decoction of the bark mixed with other herbs is especially useful for skin problems such as eczema, skin eruptions, or pimples; in mixtures of bath herbs as a detergent and astringent; in hair rinses for its curative effect on dandruff and other scalp disorders. Friend Annie has found that her lifelong scalp infection is kept in better control with a decoction of Birch bark than with any topical medicine that her doctors have ever given her. This bark is very useful in all sorts of lotions, rinses, creams, for the hair, face, or body. The dried and powdered leaves or twigs of the Birch have been successfully used for chaffed skin. Birch oil mixed with vegetable oils is useful as a hair tonic or mild antiseptic massage or body oil. **Birch leaf** drunk as a tea is a gentle sedative especially mixed with Lemon Verbena leaves. It is also used externally in baths.

Bittersweet (*Solanum dulcamara*) is used as an alterative tea as well as a water infusion for all types of skin eruptions, both internally and externally.

Blackberry leaves (*Rubus villosus, R. fructicosus*) as well as the fruits are used in facials, masks, lotions, and steams for their curative and astringent effects. The fruit is especially nice mixed with yogurt or sour cream, either eaten or applied to oily skin. The decoction works to clear and clean up blemishes, blackheads, scabby itchy scalps, and scalds. It works equally well internally for diarrhea and as a blood "cleanser."

Black currant (*Ribes nigrum*) The leaves are used as diuretic tea, diaphoretic bath, or a cool and cleansing skin lotion. These leaves have a savory use as a delicious, cooling tea. Cosmetically, an infusion of Black Currant leaves with Gum Arabic can be used as an acid antiseptic mucilage or with Quince seed as a mucilage. The entire plant belongs to the planet Jupiter. The berries are called Quinsy berries.

Bladderwrack (*Fucus vesiculosis*) as well as other Kelps and Seaweeds is great in the bath and provides various minerals and salts that cleanse and refresh the skin. It is used internally as a tea and externally as a wash to treat psoriasis. The gooey inner substance of the floats (a hollow vesicle found in certain algae containing gases and serving to buoy up the plant) mixed with a bit of rubbing alcohol and shaken up is used as a massage for cellulite and for sprains and bruises. This weed can also be mashed and bruised and used externally as a cold compress or poultice.

Borage (*Borago officinalis*) is used fresh in an infusion, as an eyewash, and as a compress for headaches. It is said to be the famous Nepenthe of Homer that will cause complete forgetfulness. When mixed with Mugwort and Parsley, it is thought to increase clairvoyance.

Bougainvillea (*glabra* and other species) The beautiful Bougainvillea, native to Central America, is one of the wonderful memoristic plants of my childhood; we used the bracts as a tea to relieve coughs but hardly ever in cosmetics.

Box (*Buxus sempervirens*) leaves and bark are used as a hair rinse for growth and as a brownish-red hair dye, especially nice when mixed with a bit of Henna.

Broom (*Cytissus scoparium*) also called Scotch Broom. The flowers are used in hair rinses for their yellow color to lighten and brighten hair; an infusion in oil is used as a massage oil for sore muscles and especially for cellulite; an infusion is used as a compress or fomentation for cellulite especially after taping; also for hand and foot soaking to relieve congested tissue.

Broomrape (*Orobanche Americana*) is a parasite on the Broom, the juice being an old remedy for clearing the skin of all sorts of blemishes, including freckles.

Buckwheat (*Fagopyrum esculentum*) flour when combined with water as a dough makes an excellent tissue-strengthening mask—very cleansing and stimulating. The flour mixed with milk, yogurt, or buttermilk instead of water is used as a galactogogue (milk increaser) when nursing. Buckwheat, however, is one of those plants that causes occasional allergic reactions, so if those delicious Buckwheat pancakes with maple syrup cause indigestion it might be sensible for you not to put it on your face. Buckwheat acts as an acid astringent and the herbal infusion is often used locally for strep (streptococcal) skin infections such as erysipelas. Buckwheat also contains rutin, an active principle of the flavenoids or vitamin P (P for permeability) which works with vitamin C.

Burdock (*Arctium lappa*) root is used in the bath as a diaphoretic; as a decoction for surface blemishes, scaly skin; in facial steams, as it affects both the oil and sweat glands; and in combinations with other herbs such as Comfrey and the licorice herbs (Licorice, Anise, and Fennel) to restore skin tone and smoothness. The leaves are used externally, as an infusion or poultice, for puffiness, bruises, or sore or tired feet. An infusion or tincture of Burdock seeds is used for skin problems. A beverage tea, made from any part of the plant, especially with other herbs such as Comfrey and Sarsaparilla, is extremely cleansing and is used for all skin problems, especially eczema. This is one of the most important cosmetic plants and should be used regularly as a beverage.

Buttercup (*Ranunculus bulbosus*) It is said that in the old days beggars used the juice of the fresh plant to produce ugly sores on their bodies so that they could beg alms from more fortunate souls.

Cacao (*Theobroma cacao*) The seeds or beans of the chocolate tree are ground up and about half become the cosmetic ingredient Cocoa butter. This fat—which smells like chocolate—is used extensively in ointments, creams, and lotions as a super emollient that softens and protects chapped hands, lips, dry skin; softens pregnant skin and helps to erase stretch marks; aids in the treatment of skin irritations; and, with other ingredients, is used to soften and erase wrinkles particularly those occurring on the neck (called turkey neck), around the eyes, and at the cor-

ners of the mouth. Mixed with coconut oil and other
vegetable oils it makes a superior skin-softening suntan lotion.

Cactus flowers (*Cactus grandiflorus, Selenicereus grandiflorus*) are occasionally used in cosmetics for their
perfume. Night-blooming Cereus blooms last about
six hours, have a heavy vanilla-type smell, and must be
picked promptly. Other Cactus flowers are more delicate and can be picked, and dropped into oil or alcohol to make a massage liquid.

Cade, oil of (*Juniperus oxycedrus*) also called Juniper tar
oil, has been used for ages in ointments and salves
for chronic eczema and minor skin problems. When
applied, it itches like crazy but also kills a bad itch.
Follow with a soothing oil or Aloe rub.

Cajuput, oil of (*Malaleuca leucadendron,* var. *minor,* or
var. *cajeputi*) is used externally for psoriasis, other
skin affections, and as a rub for sore, aching muscles.
A drop on a piece of cotton placed near the eye is
useful to relieve eyestrain and headache.

Calamus root (*Acorus calamus, Calamus aromaticus*) is a
delicious-smelling botanical used extensively in potpourris and sachets as the main scent or fixative. Small
bits are chewed to clear the voice, strengthen the
throat, and kill the taste for tobacco. It is powdered
and often mixed with Orris root and sprinkled in the
hair as a dry shampoo; or used to scent snuff, face
powders, or toothpowders. The volatile oil is obtained
by steam distillation and is used in perfumery, inhalation therapy (for the nerves, headache, hypochon-
dria), and as a scent for body and massage oil. Has
carcinogenic properties.

Camellia (the fragrant type from China or Japan is desired, *Camellia sasanqua*) flower infusion is used as a
sweet-smelling rinse for the hair. The leaves are occasionally mixed with tea to add a pleasant fragrance.

Extraction of the oil of the flowers with solvents is said to be practiced in China for perfumery purposes. Camellia seed oil is used in cooking.

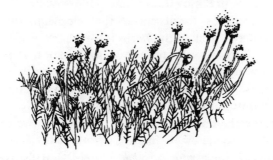

Camomile is that wonderful yellow daisy-like flower used for everything in cosmetics. However, several species are used and confused. (*Matricaria chamomilla,* German or Hungarian Camomile, produces a blue oil called azulene. This Camomile is used in medicine. *Anthemus nobilis,* Roman or English Camomile, is also called English mat Camomile.) When you buy this herb at the herb store, ask for yellow, or Hungarian, Camomile if you want to use the flower as an internal or external tea or cosmetic; and ask for the white, or Roman, type if you want the big white puffy heads for potpourris. The herb man will probably know what you want. In addition, the yellow Camomile smells sweet and appley and is called Manzanilla in Spanish countries. The root is used for toothache. An infusion used externally on the face or as a facial steam will reduce puffiness of the skin and cleanse the pores of impurities; it also helps to strengthen the tissues. The Egyptians had great reverence for the Camomile and used it in massage oils to remove aches and pains and for aching muscles. It was one of the favored strewing herbs of the Middle Ages. As a compress for the eyes it helps to brighten them and relieve weariness. In the bath it acts as a mild diaphoretic. As a thick poultice, it is used on the face and body for external swellings and will reduce pain of inflammation and neuralgia. Mixed with Poppy flowers and pods, it is also effective as a compress for abscess. A thick decoction or a hot powdered pack of the herbs is used as a rinse or hair dye. Naturally the lighter-colored your hair is, the yellower will be the effect of the herb pack on it. My hair is quite dark and a thick decoction of Camomile will only supply bright highlights; when mixed with Henna, half and half, it gives my hair a dark reddish color with yellow highlights.

Camphor (*Cinnamomum camphora*) is occasionally used in cosmetics, especially massage-type products, for its strong aromatic penetrating odor. It is slightly antiseptic and is useful as a topical application for cold sores or chapped lips, as it numbs the peripheral nerves. It is absorbed by the subcutaneous tissue; eases muscle aches and strains; and clears the head of sinus congestion and sometimes headaches. It is usually employed in conjunction with menthol. However, once when working with Camphor and experimenting with its use in various products, I inhaled it over a period of almost an hour and got a severe headache that lasted well into the night and caused me to lose sleep. So a mild sniff will clear the head but a prolonged sniff does just the opposite.

Caraway (*Carum carvi*) is occasionally used in facial steaming and is taken as an infusion by persons of pale complexion to give them a ruddy glow. A poultice of the seeds is also helpful to reduce inflammation and bruises. It has been extensively employed in love potions throughout the ages.

Cardamom (*Elettaria cardamomum*) seed is chewed to sweeten the breath and used in love potions for its sweet aromatic scent.

♧ **Carnation** (*Dianthus caryophyllus*) flowers have a sweet and spicy scent. Oil of Carnation is often made up solely of synthetic eugenol, which is a constituent of Clove oil and is used regularly by perfumers. The Carnation flower, itself, is a fragrant and tasty addition to white wines (I generally use German white wines), or champagne, and this flower wine acts as an aphrodisiac for some; for others, however, it just makes a delicious drink. The flowers soaked in vinegar and the resulting scent inhaled is useful for easing a headache; the flower or essential oil also acts in this manner. An oil made from the flowers acts on skin problems that result from nerves. Carnation massage oil (made from Carnations and not poor synthetic oils) is excellent for sore muscles and for enfleurage of a pregnant abdomen.

♧ **Carob** (*Ceratonia siliqua*, also called St. John's bread) seeds are occasionally used by public speakers or singers; they are chewed to clear the throat and clear the voice.

Carrot (*Daucus carota*) is useful lightly cooked and mashed in its own water as an excellent antiseptic mask for the face that might even provide vitamin A to the skin. A Carrot poultice is also effective on sores and skin ulcers. Mashed Carrots can be added to homemade soaps, or to a bit of honey as an excellent cleanser.

Cascarilla (*Croton eleuterea, C. eluteria*) is a scented bark used in incense and occasionally as a decoction for a skin lotion.

♧ **Cashews** (*Anacardium occidentale*) ground and mashed with buttermilk or yogurt make a mild exfoliant and beauty mask. Cashew oil is used to remove corns, warts, and other types of skin afflictions. However, it is said that the fumes of the roasting nuts can cause inflammation, and external poisoning of the face and hands. Mrs. Grieve also mentions that acid components of the Cashew nut can be used as a hair dye.

🜍 **Cassia** (*Cinnamomum cassia*) is used as a substitute for Cinnamon in cooking and incense and is also used in hair rinses and hair dyes for its wonderful scent and brown color. It is mildly astringent as a decoction. The oil is employed as a germicide. The bark is crushed and used in potpourri.

🜍 **Cassie** (*Acacia farnesiana*) See Acacia.

🜍 **Castor Oil** (*Ricinus communis*) is used externally as a lotion for skin problems and itches, rubbed into the eyebrows to help them to lie flat and shine, rubbed into the skin along the eyelashes to stimulate growth. When it is rubbed into the skin it occasionally has a laxative effect. It is used in soapmaking—in transparent soaps—and also as a nondrying oil for dry skin or rubbed into the breasts as a galactogogue.

Catnip (*Nepeta cataria*) is useful drunk as a tea for nervousness, headache, colds, or hysteria; the infusion is useful for swellings, especially mixed with black tea and placed under the eyes in the mornings for those who wake up with swollen eyes or bags, and the herb is also included with others such as Wintergreen or Gobernadora for dandruff and scalp disorders.

Cedar Various species of *Cedrus, Thuja,* and *Juniperus* are used in the bath for their tonic stimulating effect on the skin. The scent of these trees is highly aromatic and deliciously intoxicating to the senses. The *Cedrus libani* is the 1000-year-old Bible tree. Cedar leaf oil comes from *Thuja occidentalis,* which is also called the Yellow Cedar and is used directly on warts; mixed with Olive oil, it is applied externally for skin eruptions. Thuja bark and needles are used in baths for their mentally relaxing and tonic effect. They are slightly astringent and especially good in the morning bath for their stimulating effect on the muscles. The oil is used in soapmaking and is very aromatic

(Caswell-Massey sells a Thuja soap called Fenjal Soap).

Cédrat oil (*Citrus medica*, var. *bajoura*) See Citron.

⚘ **Celandine** (*Chelidonium majus*), dried and mixed with other herbs such as Comfrey, is used in baths; the fresh juice has been applied directly on warts, ring-worm, and corns, but great care should be exercised that the juice does not get onto any other part of the skin as it can act as an irritant; in an ointment or mixed with sulphur it helps to cure skin problems such as eczema; a decoction eases the itch of itchy places.

Celery (*Apium graveolens*) tops are useful in all sorts of creams and lotions or facial steams; they act as a tonic on the skin, especially to give tone to older skin. I know of no use in cosmetics for Celery seeds.

Centaury (*Erythraea centaurium*) lotion is useful to remove freckles, marks, and spots on the skin.

Cereus See Cactus.

Cherry (*Prunus virginiana*) bark is used in herb mixtures as a hair-conditioning rinse for ease in combing. It is especially effective mixed with Ragwort and Nettle.

Chickweed (*Stellaria media*) is a demulcent used in lotions and salves for skin problems and also as a poultice for sores or abscesses. Effective also in bath herbs.

Chrysanthemums of many species are used in herbal hair rinses and hair packs as a dye plant. (See also Marigold.)

Cicely, Sweet (*Myrrhis odorata*, sometimes called the myrrh plant) is a nice addition to waters and lotions for its aromatic scent. It is a mild cleanser of old wounds, and the essence is said to act as an aphrodisiac.

Cinnamon (*Cinnamomum zeylanicum*) is used in cosmetics for its aromatic and astringent qualities. It makes a nice addition to hair rinses, imparts a slight brown tone, and is mixed with Indigo to soften the black and scent the hair or with Henna to soften the red. Cinnamon is also much used in incense and potpourri; an infusion is useful as a wash for wounds or skin problems.

🔥**Cinquefoil** (*Potentilla reptans*) also called Five-Finger Grass, is normally used dried in bath herbs as an astringent; the infusion is used as an eye lotion to soothe the eyes; as a gargle for sore throat; as a mouthwash for sore gums.

Citron (*Citrus medica*) also called the Cédrat, is a fruit whose essential oil is used in perfumery. However, Parry's *Cyclopedia of Perfumery* states that the Cédrat oil of commerce is usually a mixture of Lemon with other citrus oils. French "oil of Cédrat" is, when pure, Citron oil, and French "oil of Citron" is oil of Lemon. It's all wonderfully confusing, *n'est-ce pas?*

Citronella (*Cymbopogon nardus*) grass is also called Lemon Balm but it is not the Lemon Balm known as *Melissa officinalis*. This fragrant grass oil is often used in insect repellants as it repels mosquitoes and other bugs. The essential oil is used as a raw material in the manufacture of other oils such as geraniol, and when creating synthetic oils of Linden, Lily of the Valley, Carnation, Rose, or other floral scents. Oil of Citronella is also used extensively in soapmaking. The finest quality obtained by steam distillation comes from Java but it is also manufactured in Ceylon. Citronella grass is excellent as a wash for oily conditions of the skin, is a normalizer of the sebaceous glands, and is used in hair rinses to give the hair a lustrous sheen. Some use the oil in aromatherapy as a heart stimulant.

Civet leaves are probably the dried leaves of Chives, which is called in French *Ail Civitte*. While examining an herb store catalog some time ago, I came across the entry "Civet leaves" and proceeded to order two pounds. The green objects arrived, and their smell was musky and somewhat unpleasant. So I wrote to the company and asked what the generic name of their Civet leaves was, and they responded it was *Civettictus civetta,* which I knew to be the name of the civet cat and had absolutely nothing to do with plants. I wrote back to them with this information, and they responded that they did not know what their Civet leaves were, which started me on a two-year search into this seeming mystery; the result is that I found Civet leaves are probably identical with Chives. But who knows? If you have any information about Civet leaves, please correspond with me in San Francisco. Chives are rich in sulphur and therefore very useful in hair rinses for scalp problems. For a hair rinse, mix the dried or freshly cut up Chives with Ambrette seeds and maybe a bit of ground-up Cinnamon for astringency.

Clary Sage (*Salvia sclarea*) oil is obtained by distillation and is an important fixative in perfumery. In addition it has the special property of toning other scents and alleviating their harshness. It is used in many colognes, toilet waters, powders, soaps, perfumes, sachets, potpourris, and many other cosmetics. It blends with the other herbal scents, especially Rosemary and Bergamot, but also Lavender, Musk, and Chypre. The dried herb is used in baths as an aromatic astringent and, mixed with Lemon Verbena, it makes a particularly nice warming bath or lotion to cleanse the face. The seeds as a decoction are used to clear the eyes of foreign substances.

Clivers (*Galium aparine*) or Cleavers, is used as a wash for skin diseases—including psoriasis—as well as for mild burns, sunburns, and freckles.

Clove (*Eugenia caryophyllus, E. caryophyllata, Caryophyllus aromaticus*) The dried flower buds are chewed for bad breath, used in bath herb mixtures as an astringent, antiseptic, aromatic, and in herbal hair rinses for brown or red hair. Clove is also a wonderfully fragrant addition to all sorts of cosmetic waters and lotions; as a mouthwash; in aromatherapy for sleep, to relieve melancholy, to aid the eyes and memory; in potpourris and sachets—especially with rose-type scents. The essential oil obtained by distillation is a powerful antiseptic, used in carious teeth to allay pain. It is effective in perfumery as a fixative or as a part of synthetic oil of Carnation as well as in other synthetic essential oils.

Clover, Red (*Trifolium pratense*) is useful in all sorts of cosmetics—especially in facial steams, bath herb mixtures, hair rinses, and other shampoos—as an alterative and cleanser. It is also used as a wash for skin problems and pimples. As a thick poultice, it is used for the athlete's foot fungus.

Cochineal (*Dactylopius coccus*) is a beetle used in cosmetics as a red dye.

Cocoa See Cacao.

Coltsfoot (*Tussilago farfara*) can be used externally as a poultice for welts and swellings. Eyes can be bathed with an infusion of the flowers in hot water.

Columbine (*Aquilegia vulgaris*) seeds can be mashed and simmered in Olive oil to rub into aching joints or into the scalp to repel lice.

Comfrey (*Symphytum officinale*) is one of the most useful plants in herbal cosmetics or medicine. Both the fresh and dried root and leaf can be used. In the *Physician's Desk Reference* (1970, p. 956), it states that "allantoin [Comfrey's active ingredient] has been reported to liquefy pus and necrotic protein thus accelerating debridement of lesions and denuded areas." It is a cell proliferant and cell regenerative and, with continuous use, regenerates aging tissues. Comfrey can be used in lotions, creams, salves, ointments, vaginal douches,

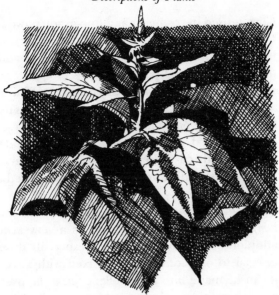

COMFREY

hair rinses and shampoos, hand creams, massage or body oils, and just about anything else you can think of. It is both emollient (demulcent) and astringent. Incredibly easy to grow, it will thrive most anywhere. I have it in a shady corner of my yard near the musk rose, where it gets up to three feet high and bears bluish-purple flowers most of the summer (here in San Francisco, summer is cool, wet, and foggy). It is especially valuable in bath herb mixtures, and I would count it as one of the five most valuable and useful herbs in my medicine and cosmetic cabinet. (The other four would be Mint, Lavender, Echinacea, and Garlic.)

Corn (*Zea mays*—Indian corn) oil is used in cosmetics for normal to oily skin but I cannot recommend its use since a large percentage of the pesticides and fungicides that are employed in this country are used on the corn and cotton crops. Corn silk from red Indian

Corn is used in cosmetics as a fine-grade powder and face powder that is a soothing emollient. Cornmeal is used in soapmaking for cleansing; also as an addition to masks and facial packs.

Cornflower (*Centaurea cyanus*) also called the Blue Bottle and sometimes Bachelor Button. The flower is used in hair rinses for pale blond, white, or gray hair. It can also be applied as a thick pack on the hair for deeper color. The dried flowers are used in potpourris for color. A distilled water from the petals is used as an eyewash.

Costmary (*Chrysanthemum balsamita, Pyrethrum tanacetum*) also called the Bible Leaf, is a very aromatic addition to creams and lotions—especially those for normal to oily complexions. Mixed with Lavender, it can be made into an excellent facial oil, useful in acneic conditions. Also a good massage oil. Dried, it is excellent in potpourris and sachets.

Cowslip (*Primula veris*) is the flower mentioned in *A Midsummer Night's Dream,* purported to have a special and magical value for the complexion. And, indeed, it is useful in all sorts of cosmetics and hair products for both oily and dry complexions—especially skin on the dry side. The flowers are used as a wash for pimples, spots, sunburn, and wrinkles. Distilled water of Cowslips is used as a mild astringent; the powdered flowers with Oatmeal or Cornmeal make a good scrub. These powdered flowers mixed with talcum and Camomile also make an excellent body powder.

Creosote bush (*Larrea divaricata, L. Mexicana*) also called Gobernadora and Chapparal, is used primarily as a hair tonic to relieve itchy scalp and cure dandruff. It is used as a wash to disinfect and deodorize the body, but since it is so highly aromatic and unpleasant to some, it is best used mixed with other more pleasantly scented herbs such as Peppermint.

Cuckoopint (*Arum vulgare, A. maculatum*) picked, dried, aged, and powdered has been used in the past as a face powder, starch, wrinkle remover, and poultice for sores, swellings, and ringworm.

Cucumber (*Cucumis sativus*) is one of those plants incredibly useful in all types of cosmetics. The juice is used in many different kinds of creams, lotions, sunburn preparations, soaps, masks, and packs as a cooling, soothing, and healing substance. It is very useful for freckles, cutaneous eruptions, or irritated skin. Direct application of sliced Cucumbers is helpful for irritated eyes or to soothe a windburn. Cucumber can be mixed with Glycerin, Elder water, Orange water, Rosewater, with tincture of Benzoin or salicylic acid added as a preservative. Cucumber jelly, a mucilage of Gum Tragacanth or Quince seed with Cucumber water instead of water, is excellent as an aftershave. Cucumber ointment is especially good for wrinkles, skin bleaching, or softening hardened skin. Essence of Cucumber is used in the blending of some perfumes and concentrated Cucumber perfume can be made by repeated extraction and distillation.

Cumin (*Cuminum cyminum*) oil is often used in perfumery.

Curry plant (a species of *Helichrisum*) has a Lavender-like leaf and a yellow button-like flower like the Yarrow. If you gently rub the plant it smells like a Curry powder. The flower can be used in hair rinses and packs for light or blond hair.

Cyclamens (*Cyclamen spp.*) are occasionally used as a cosmetic wash to soften the skin and clear it of marks.

Daffodil (*Narcissus spp.*) flowers are occasionally infused in oil to make massage and body oils useful for the soothing effect of the scent and to relax the nervous system.

Daisy (*Bellis perennis*) flowers are used externally in lotions for skin disease, wounds, and bruises.

Dandelion (*Taraxacum spp.*) greens are very high in vitamin A and, in fact, contain more of this substance than Carrots and Apricots. They are useful in facial steams, facial packs, as a wash for eczema and other skin complaints, in bath herbs, infused in oil as a bath or body oil. Dandelions are a specific for the liver and thus are one of the most useful herbs in the home cosmetic cabinet. Dandelion tea—one ounce infused in two cups of boiling water for five to ten minutes, strained and honeyed—drunk throughout the day is a useful addition to your external cosmetic treatments.

Deer Tongue (*Frasera speciosa, Liatris odoratissima*) is used in bath herbs because of its sweet aromatic scent which is due to its coumarin contents. It is also used in herbal smoking mixtures.

Dill (*Anethum graveolens*) oil and herb are used in soap-making. The essential oil is also used in aromatherapy.

Dittany of Crete (*Origanum dictamnus*) is indigenous to Crete; the leaf infusion has been used to ease the pain of difficult labor and also for gastric distress; bracts and flowers are drunk as a pleasant relaxing tea; three leaves are chewed every few hours for sore throat pain; the leaves mixed with Parsley, Garlic, Thyme, salt, and Pepper make an interesting fish sauce; a salve of the root is used for sciatica pain; the leaves infused in oil make a useful massage oil for the legs and hips. The distilled water is an excellent cosmetic for all types and conditions of skin.

Dock (all varieties: *Rumex alpinus*—Herb Patience; *R. crispus*—Yellow Dock, used for the skin and the liver) is a mild astringent and detergent and is used in bath herbs and in facial washes for skin eruptions or diseases or freckles. Dock contains more vitamin A than Carrots but less than Dandelions. Infusions of

Dock are used as cleansing mouthwashes for the gums and teeth and powdered Dock root is used as a dentifrice.

Dragon's Blood (*Dracaena spp., Daemonorops draco*) is used to color tooth powders, and it also acts as an astringent. There is a fine specimen of this tree in the Huntington Gardens of Los Angeles.

Echinacea (*E. augustifolia*) root is one of the most useful herbs for the home medicinal chest. It also has great use in cosmetics, mainly as an internal cleanser for skin conditions. I normally take it in gelatin capsule form because the tea tastes somewhat unpleasant.

Elder (*Sambucus canadensis, S. nigra*) leaf water or ointment is used for cooling and softening the skin. Elderberries boiled in wine or vinegar make a black hair dye. Elder flowers are the most useful part of the Elder tree in cosmetics and generally are distilled into Elder flower water, which is used as a healing and gentle astringent for dry or normal skin. They have a sweet scent and are occasionally used in perfumery. Elder flower water or tea made at home is used as a wash to cleanse the skin and clear the complexion of freckles, or as an eyewash, or to ease a sunburn. Mixed with salt or with Glycerin and borax, it is used for eruptions. Elder flowers are also added to bath water to ease irritable skin or nerves; mixed with Peppermint and Yerba Santa, it is a fine diaphoretic tea to take for a cold; steeped in oil, it makes a relaxing and soothing bath and massage oil. Elder face cream is an excellent day- or night-time application.

Elecampane (*Inula helenium*) is occasionally used as a wash for skin disease, but it is best mixed with other facial herbs such as Comfrey plus an aromatic. Also added to bath water.

Elm (*Ulmus campestris*) bark and leaves are used in baths or distilled into a water that is useful for skin eruptions and cutaneous diseases. It is slightly astringent and emollient.

Elm, Slippery (*Ulmus fulva*) is demulcent and emollient and is very useful in herbal practice. It is healing, soothing, and, when taken internally, strengthening. It is usually purchased in powder form and, as such, makes a fine poultice for all types of skin afflictions—wounds, abscesses, sores, inflamed surfaces, ulcerous sores, burns, boils, and skin diseases. A poultice also reduces pain (it would improve the poultice to add Comfrey root in a ratio of 1:1).

Eucalyptus (*E. spp.*, *E. globulus* is the common Eucalyptus used as an antiseptic; *E. citriodora*—lemon-scented— is used in perfumery; *E. odorata* is used in soapmaking) leaves are used in bath herbs for the antiseptic action and are especially nice when you have a cold or other respiratory problem (the aromatic scent coming from the bath water seems to clear the respiratory passages). The leaves are also used in sleep pillows for asthma or bronchial troubles, and they are useful in mixtures of herbs for dandruff or scalp conditions. The aromatic oil, especially from the lemon-scented Eucalyptus, is used in soapmaking, for massage or bath oils, and also in ointments for skin affections. It is also used in many over-the-counter preparations. Mixed with oil and solidified with beeswax, this ointment is very good for chapped hands, and as a rub for aching joints or muscles.

Eyebright (*Euphrasia officinalis*) is used as a wash for sore or puffy eyes.

Fennel (*Foeniculum vulgare*) seed, ground, is used in facial steams to medicate the pores, and Fennel oil is used in perfumery and for scenting soaps. An infusion of Fennel with a bit of Eyebright makes a soothing eyewash and is said to have a strengthening effect on the eyes; an infusion of Fennel seed and Nettle leaves makes a useful tea for those who wish to lose weight, and it is also a galactogogue.

Fenugreek (*Trigonella foenum-graecum*) seeds, sprouted, are an excellent *addition* to the diet for diabetic and arthritic afflictions. Fenugreek apparently contains B_{12}, organic iron, and a hormone that makes it an excellent tea for vegetarians. A poultice of Fenugreek seeds is emollient and, therefore, useful to relieve boils or abscess.

Ferns are generally used in herbal medicine and have very little use in herbal cosmetics, except for the *Maidenhair Fern* (*Asplenium trichomanes*), which has an old reputation as an excellent hair wash to stimulate growth and prevent the hair from falling out, and, mixed with Camomile and infused in oil, for swellings and for drying up moist sores. Powdered roots of *Bracken Fern* (*Pteris aquilina*) are used as an astringent to dry up old sores. The root of the *Common Polypody* (*Polypodium vulgare*) is used as a tonic tea to help in the healing of skin diseases. The root of the *Kings Fern*—also called Male Fern or Royal Fern (*Osmunda regalis*)—is very useful infused in oil as a massage oil for the lower back or as an ointment for sores and bruises.

Feverfew (also called the Febrifuge plant or *Pyrethrum parthenium*) in my garden is a nice bushy plant and keeps producing lots of aromatic flowers throughout the year that are about one inch across with white outer rays, the center round part, called the floret, being about ⅝ inch in diameter, pale yellow, and nearly flat. This is a plant often mislabeled in nurseries and should probably be ordered from one of the more reputable plant dealers such as those listed in Chapter VI. I have ordered seeds of this plant and the plant itself from five different nurseries in the

United States and have received three entirely different plants under the name of Feverfew. However,
though they look different, they smell remarkably
alike. Feverfew infused in cold water and applied to
the face makes an excellent poultice for a sensitive
face or headache. It can also be used in bath herbs or
for facial steams.

Figs (*Ficus carica*) are important in many ancient
mythologies, both in religious ceremonies and as an
aphrodisiac. Figs are mildly laxative and can be applied cosmetically as emollient and cleansing masks.
They are also useful as a poultice for swellings, sores,
or a dental abscess (use the soft mashed inner part).
Occasionally the milky stalk juice is applied directly on
warts to remove them. Mr. Freitas was one of the
mysterious people of my childhood. He lived next
door and kept pigeons and peacocks in his backyard,
stagecoaches in the barn, and at his back door an
enormous Fig tree. Whenever we walked through his
property to get to the local swimming pool, he would
appear at the back door with a yapping little dog,
offering his gorgeous Figs. I always felt I was Eve
being tempted by the Devil. I don't believe I ever ate
one of his Figs; they made me too nervous.

Figwort (*Scrophularia nodosa*) is occasionally used externally as a poultice for sores or pimples.

Filaree (*Alfilerilla spp.*) is used in herb bath mixtures for
joint aches and for rheumatism.

Flax (*Linum usitatissimum*) seed is used as a mucilage to set
hair or as an emollient and demulcent poultice. The
poultice eases pain and irritation and is commonly
used for boils, sores, and irritations. Linseed oil (the
oil from the Flax seed) is a drying oil rarely used for
oily skin and normally mixed with other oils.

Fo-ti-tieng (*Hydrocotyle asiatica minor*) is used in bath herbs
for its rejuvenating effect on the skin, especially in

conjunction with Patchouli, Comfrey, and Ginseng.

Frangipani is also called the Plumeria (*P. acuminata*) or Melia in Hawaii. *P. rubra* is the red Plumeria. See Plumeria for uses.

Frankincense (various species of *Boswellia,* especially *B. carteri*) is used as incense and occasionally in facial steams or inhalations for sore throat or laryngitis. It forms part of the eye make-up substance called kohl. There is an old recipe to remove pimples that uses Frankincense: Boil an egg, separate the white and sprinkle over it powdered Frankincense, put it away in a cool place until the white liquefies, and then apply this to the pimples or the acne (sounds yucky to me!).

Fuchsia (*Zauschneria* or *Fuchsia californica*) flowers dried and powdered are used to dust on wounds and sores; a wash of the fresh flowers is used as a poultice for deep sores. The dried flowers also make a nice addition to potpourri for deep red color.

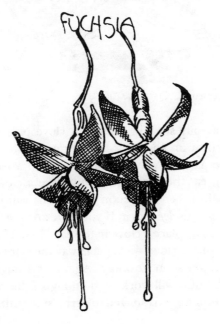

✿ **Fumitory** (*Fumaria officinalis*) is said to be used as a wash for infants' cradle cap, as a face wash to clear up freckles and acne pimples, and in soapmaking.

Gardenia (*Gardenia spp.*) tea is drunk for hysteria and applied externally for chronic skin ailments. Inhale the scent to soothe the psyche and make the flower oil by enfleurage for use as a body and massage oil.

Garlic (*Allium sativum*) The magic plant. I use it for everything and consider it one of the five most valuable medicinal or cosmetic herbs. Eaten or applied externally, it is beneficial. If you cook it, it loses most of its potent valuable qualities; it should be used absolutely

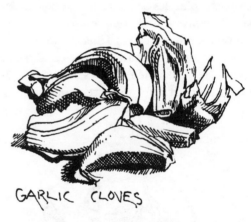

GARLIC CLOVES

fresh or only slightly heated. A clove placed in the mouth near an abscess will help remove the swelling and the pain. If you or your pets have worms (pinworms), eat the raw cloves and place a clove in the anus before bed and soon the worms will be gone. However, this *does* burn. If you have an earache or an infected ear, place a clove in the ear (do not break the surface of the clove—just peel away the skin), and the earache will soon go away. Again, this might burn slightly, but it will work soon enough. The raw juice mixed with water is sniffed to cure a sinus infection or an infectious runny nose (see *Herbs & Things*). The mashed cloves are applied externally for swellings and sores and dabbed on pimples and acne to cure them. However, the smell might be repugnant to some. Four or five cloves of Garlic infused in water, vinegar, or wine makes an excellent wash for the scalp to stimulate growth and clear up dandruff. Last September I planted Elephant Garlic that was harvested this August. The bulbs weighed 10–16 ounces each, each bulb having 5 or 6 cloves. This Garlic is very mild and can be thinly sliced and eaten in sandwiches; when cooked, it tastes like potatoes.

Geranium (*Geranium spp.*—the common garden Geranium) leaves are useful wherever an astringent is needed. The root of the wild Geranium is called Alum root and is often used as a vaginal douche for persistent types of discharge. Geranium flowers can be dried and used in potpourris. Our interest in Geraniums really concerns the scented types, the various species of *Pelargonium*. These plants, with their marvelously scented foliage of spice, citrus, fruit, herb, or flower, can be used in all types of cosmetic

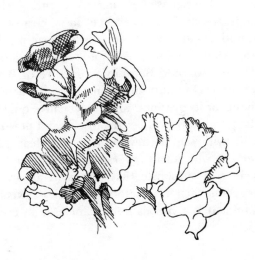

preparations. They are especially nice in facial steams, as a stimulating tea, as a mild astringent wash, in stimulating bath herbs, hair rinses, or facial masks. The foliage when dried is really nice in herby pot-pourris. Rose Geranium leaves are used in jelly, and the apple-scented Geranium is delicious in tea. Geranium oil is obtained by distillation of the leaves and stems of various species of the *Pelargonium* and is a part of many types of perfumes—especially Rose types—or as a substitute for Rose perfumes. It is also used in many cosmetics and in soapmaking.

Ginger (*Zingibar officinale*) decoction is occasionally used as a cleansing mouthwash.

Ginseng (*Panax quinquefolium*—American; *P. schinseng*—Oriental) has of late been enjoying a reputation as a super cosmetic and is used in places like Hollywood and London as a super panacea for all types of cosmetic ills. Taken internally it does work as a rejuvenative and tonic. I have found it excellent as a skin conditioner in a bath herb mixture combined with other herbs such as Comfrey and Patchouli. It is also used in skin masks and packs and makes a wonderful skin cleanser, eye mask, moisturizing lotion, or night cream. For an excellent facial cleanser and restorative make an infusion of Peppermint, Comfrey, and Alfalfa and use this liquid to make a mucilage of Tragacanth, add Benzoin or tincture of Benzoin as a preservative and some Ginseng as the active ingredient for its grittiness and rejuvenative qualities. For the pores, mix powdered Ginseng and powdered Alfalfa with sage honey, and pat on clean skin, and remove with warm water, then cool water.

Glycerin is a substance that occurs in all animal and vegetable fats; it is a colorless, odorless, sweet, syrupy liquid. It is a viscous humectant used in creams, lotions, mouthwashes, cough syrups, soapmaking, drugs, and foods. It is a useful addition to the home cosmetic maker—mixed with Rose or Orange water, it makes an excellent hand or body lotion, very effective on chapped or dry skin.

Goldenrod (*Solidago odora*) As Euell Gibbons was wont to say on television, "It makes a delicious tay." It is also aromatic and stimulating to the tissues and can be added to a facial steam for its astringent and diaphoretic qualities. These same qualities make it a nice addition to the bath, especially for oily skin, and in a shampoo or hair rinse it can give the hair nice highlights. Of course it is especially useful to those with light-colored hair. It can be used as a compress for a headache.

Golden Seal (*Hydrastis canadensis*) is an herb that may soon be unavailable because of our extensive export of it; indeed, our government agencies, seeing that it works, want to make it illegal to buy. However, it is more useful as a medicinal plant than as a cosmetic plant. The root can be used as an astringent yellow dye or hair rinse. Mixed with Comfrey root, it becomes less astringent and can therefore be used by those with dry or thin hair. It can also be used as a mouthwash for thrush or any other disordered condition of the mouth. It is used externally in all sorts of lotions for various skin conditions including acne and dandruff. The active ingredients of this plant can be absorbed through the skin, and it should be remembered that this absorption is cumulative (can be poisonous), and therefore Golden Seal should only be used for short periods of time when really necessary.

Gold Thread (*Coptis trifolia*) as an infusion with other herbs is useful as a hair rinse or dye. Since it is a potent astringent, it makes an excellent mouthwash or wash for all sorts of skin pimples, bumps, or sores. It has also been used to some extent as a mouthwash for thrush.

Gotu Kola (*Hydrocotyl asiatica*) is occasionally used in bath herb mixtures for its rejuvenating effect on the skin with Comfrey, Patchouli, and Ginseng. It is often confused with but may in fact be identical with Fo-ti-tieng.

Grapes (*Vitis vinifera*) are cooling and demulcent. They can be mashed and applied directly to the skin to make a nourishing mask. Seeds and leaves are astringent and are used in the bath as a restorative. The sap is called Lachryma and is used as a lotion for the eyes, especially weak eyes.

Groundsels also called Ragworts, are not the same as Ragweeds, which occasionally are also called Ragworts. *Senecio vulgaris* is used as a wash for the skin; *S. maritima* or Cineraria (a common garden Groundsel) is used as a compress for tired eyes; and all can be used in the bath as a mild diaphoretic.

Gypsyweed or the *Lycopus* is an astringent used in herbal steams and baths and also as a wash for many types of skin problems. It is said to be used by gypsies as a stain for the face.

Heartsease See Pansy.

Heather (*Erica vulgaris*) water, distilled from the flowers, cures inflamed eyes. An oil made from the flowers has a reputation for curing shingles and skin eruptions.

Heliotrope (*Heliotropium peruvianum*), also called Cherry Pie, is used in the home for its wonderfully fragrant scent. A tincture of the blossoms is used as a compress for headache or as a gargle for sore throat. A cold infusion of the flowers is used as a rinse for the hair or body, and a cold oil infusion can be used as a bath or body oil. In aromatherapy the scent is inhaled to soothe the nerves.

Henna (*Lawsonia alba* or *L. inermis*) is a famous Egyptian herb used for cosmetics and medicines for hundreds, nay thousands of years. It makes an excellent hair wash, rinse, or dye, depending on the strength of the solution. The powdered leaf can be mixed with other herbs to make different-colored rinses, depending on one's desires. You can stain your fingernails or dye patterns onto your body with it. The leaves used externally as a wash are helpful in clearing up all types of skin affections, and mixed with Camomile and simmered in oil, Henna makes an excellent massage oil said to make the limbs more supple. The flowers are used in massage oils, and the essence is extracted for a perfume oil.

Hibiscus (*H. rosa-sinensis*) flowers and leaves are used as a hair rinse and in facial steams as an emollient (see also Jamaica flowers).

Holly, also called the Holy Tree (*Ilex aquifolium*). The leaves, berries, and bark are all used. The leaves are a diaphoretic cosmetic and an infusion given in certain respiratory ailments. The berries are violently emetic and probably should not be used. Holly has very little cosmetic use.

Hollyhock (*Althaea rosea*) is very useful in hair rinses as an emollient dye plant especially for dark hair or white hair to get rid of the yellowish tinge. The flowers come in assorted colors, and the rather blackish blue ones, when dried, possess an interesting smell most useful in Rose potpourris. These emollient flowers are also good in herbal baths or in a compress for soothing facial dryness and softening.

Honeysuckle (*Lonicera caprifolium*) flowers are infused in oil to make an elegant massage or body oil. The distilled water is excellent as a headwash for head pain or headache and also as a wash for delicate skin. Honeysuckle flower syrup is delicious and exceedingly useful as a gargle for sore throat; it is taken

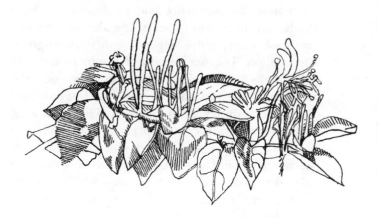

frequently for asthma. When used frequently, Honeysuckle bark oil is a good application for wrinkles.

Hops (*Humulus lupulus*) are occasionally used to yield a brown dye for the hair, and an infusion with Camomile is used to reduce swellings; this same mixture can be infused in oil as a body oil.

Horseradish (*Rorippa armoracia*) infused in oil with other herbs such as Orange peel is occasionally used as a very stimulating massage oil for aches and pains. It is a powerful stimulant and rubefacient.

Horsetails (*Equisetum arvense*) are said to make an effective wash for the hair to stimulate growth and eliminate dandruff. However, I have not used it for this purpose. The distilled water, or an infusion, is used for the face to clear up pimply breakouts.

Houseleek (*Sempervivum tectorum*) has been used for hundreds of years as a beautifying cosmetic. It is said that this plant was one of the ingredients in Ninon de Lenclos' famous herb bath formula. It also had a reputation with the ancient Greeks as an aphrodisiac. An infusion of the herb is used both internally and externally for all types of skin diseases, burns, warts, cuts, and as a wash for inflamed eyes. Very good used by

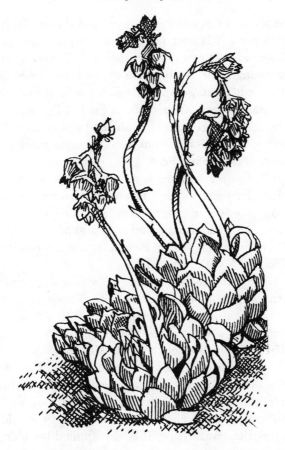

HENS 'N' CHICKENS

itself or with honey or cream in lotions, potions, facial steams, and baths. It is mainly cooling, and astringent.

Huckleberry (*Vaccinium myrtillus*) leaves and fruits are used as an external astringent application for oily skin.

Hyacinth, Grape (*Muscari spp.*) flowers are occasionally dried and used for the blue color in potpourris.

Hyssop (*Hyssopus officinalis*) is a potent diaphoretic in the bath and is especially nice when used absolutely fresh. However, it is best mixed with Thyme, Mint, and Rosemary. It can also be used as a cleansing facial steaming herb. An infusion of the leaves in oil is an excellent massage application for aching limbs and rheumatic pains. Hyssop oil is used in liquors (chartreuse). The scent can be inhaled by persons of hysterical disposition to calm them. In other times it was used as a strewing herb.

🕱 **Indigo** (*Indigofera tinctoria*) is a plant from which a blue-black dye extracted by fermentation is used in writing inks, as a dyestuff for the hair, and, well diluted, as a rinse. The color can be altered by adding other herbs: Clove for a rich brown, Henna for a reddish cast (see Chapter XVII).

Iris (*Iris florentina*—Orris root; *I. foetidissima*—Stinking Iris; *I. pseudacorus*—Yellow Iris; *I. versicolor*—Blue Flag) furnishes the famous Orris root, which is an important cosmetic (see Orris). A decoction of the dried root of the foetid or Stinking Iris is used as a cleansing wash for facial eruptions. An infusion of the Yellow Iris is used as a hair rinse. Iris flowers infused in oil can be used as a massage oil for aching legs or, during pregnancy, for muscle cramps (it is said to strengthen weak legs). It is also applied for blemish control as a daily wash.

Irish Moss (*Chondrus crispus*), a sea plant, contains a substance called Carrageen that is used as a suspending and emulsifying agent in cosmetics, especially creams, and in antiwrinkle preparations. It is a soothing emollient, especially useful for dry or aging skin problems.

Ivy (*Hedera helix*) is used in mixtures of bath herbs for the nerves and muscles. In old books it is also recommended as a sunburn remover when boiled in sweet butter and applied.

🕱 **Ivy** (*Glechoma hederacea*—Ground Ivy) is used in bath

herbs for problem skin and is especially useful mixed with Camomile, Comfrey, Yarrow, and other like herbs.

🐢 **Jaborandi** *(Pilocarpus jaborandi)* has an especial reputation as a stimulant to hair growth. It contains pilocarpine and is terribly dangerous if taken internally. In all my classes I emphasize over and over the importance of testing herbs for strength when they are used internally, that one must test every new batch of herbs by making a very weak tea and gradually increasing the dosage until one finds the proper effective strength because each batch is of variable strength, stronger or weaker than the last. However, when I decided to take some Jaborandi tea to help me lose weight (body water) quickly for an upcoming physical, I stupidly ignored my own advice of moderation and took a quantity of Jaborandi, ground up and stuffed into gelatin capsules, that was much too powerful. The first symptom occurred 20 minutes after I took the dose and was in bed; I started to perspire and salivate so profusely that I was afraid I would choke on my own saliva, and so I sat up. Then I took a towel to sponge my body and to soak up the saliva and water that was pouring out of every orifice. I wrapped myself in blankets and made some extra strong black tea to counteract the effects of the overdose of Jaborandi. Within 2 hours I was able to go to bed again safely; in the morning my pillow was so soaked with perspiration that I was able to wring it out and when I weighed myself I found that I had lost over 5 pounds in 3 hours. A much too dangerous way to lose weight!

Cosmetically, Jaborandi is used in shampoos and herbal hair rinses, hair tonics and lotions to stimulate the pores, and occasionally in baths to get rid of excess water in the tissues; it is also useful as a wash for skin problems such as psoriasis.

Jamaica flowers (Several species of *Hibiscus*—one of the nicest is *H. sabdariffa* from Mexico) are used wherever an astringent herb is indicated in cosmetics. It also makes a delicious tea to drink. The red flowers can be used to color hair red.

Jasmine (*Jasminum officinale*—common White Jasmine; *J. odoratissimum*—true Yellow Jasmine from the Canary Islands; *J. sambac*—to scent tea; *J. Grandiflorum*—Spanish Jasmine) flowers can be used in many ways in cosmetic preparations. The flowers infused in a fine oil have been used as a massage oil to overcome frigidity; this same oil added to the bath is excellent for smoothing the skin. Jasmine flowers added to white wine (German white wines or champagne seem to work the best) make an excellent and tasty drink that is said to act as an aphrodisiac. Essential oil of Jasmine is inhaled to relax the body, facilitate childbirth (I used it for this), and in sleep pillows to help one fall asleep. This oil is obtained by the enfleurage method and is becoming increasingly expensive. The flowers are wonderful with Rose and Comfrey when added to the bath, and in facial steams to smooth and cleanse the skin. Mrs. Grieve states that boiled leaves of the Eastern Jasmine are "used to anoint the head for complaints of the eye, and an oil obtained from the roots is used medicinally to arrest the secretion of milk."

Jewelweed (*Impatiens biflora*) juice is used externally to relieve poison oak irritation, and other species are said to be used for dying the fingernails red or as a hairwash.

Jonquil (*Narcissus jonquilla*) Jonquil flowers, or their essential oil, are used in perfumery and, when inhaled, influence the nervous system and work on the senses. They have also been used in the treatment of hysteria. The fresh flowers when displayed in any quantity in a room can cause nausea and headache in sensitive people. The flowers are also said to be a potent remedy for some skin diseases of a pustular nature.

Juniper (*Juniperus communis*) berries are used in baths for aching muscles, and the oil is used in soapmaking and in massage or in bath oils and liniments.

Kale (*Brassica oleracea*, var. *acephala*) as well as all the other members of the cabbage family is used cosmetically as a wash for sore or bloodshot eyes.

Kelp (a general name for large brown Seaweeds) is used internally as a food supplement for its vitamins and minerals, which are beneficial to the skin, fingernails, and hair. It can be used with positive effects in weight control diets and can be added to the bath for smoothing the skin.

"The Indians of Sitka, Alaska, make use of the tube-like stipes of bull kelp as an instrument for treating earache; the thin end of the kelp is placed in the ear and the bulb is put on a hot, wet stone, thereby allowing the steam to enter and soothe the auditory canal. Seaweeds are also used for poultices for bruises and cuts."—Gloria Dunstan, *Seaweeds*. Kelp makes excellent soil fertilizer and can be spread about without preparation and then plowed into the ground as a source of potash. Kelp is a term used for many species of the Seaweed Fucus (see also Seaweed). It was the original source of iodine, being discovered by Courtois in 1812. Iodine does not occur in nature in the uncombined state but is widely distributed in sea water, some Seaweeds, and various mineral and medicinal springs. Kelp has *alterative* properties and reduces obesity by its action on the thyroid. It is also used in chronic psoriasis. (The recommended dosage is 25 grams of Kelp extract before each of 3 meals a day, which seems like a lot to me.)

Kings Fern See Ferns.

🜚 **Kohl** is a black powder containing a number of ingredi-
    ents, including Frankincense and, it is thought, lead
    and antimony. Consequently, Kohl can cause eye
    irritation, madness, and blindness. Some artificial
    Kohls are made and sold in this country to be used
    in the same way as the original (that is, as an eye
    make-up).

Labdanum (*Cistus ladaniferus*) See also Rock Rose. The
    essential oil, steam-distilled from this gum, is called
    Cistus oil or oil of Ciste. Cistus oil can also be obtained
    by steam distillation from the leaves and tops.

Lady's Mantle (*Alchemilla vulgaris*) is used for sleep and
    also, when infused in water or oil, as a massage for
    hanging breasts; it is thought to cause the breasts to
    grow smaller and more firm. It is used in bath herbs
    for sore, inflamed skin and acts as an astringent.

🜚 **Laurel** (*Laurus nobilis*) berry oil is used in perfumery and in
    liniments for aching muscles, bruises, and sprains.
    The leaves are employed in baths for rheumatism and
    aching, overworked muscles.

Lavender (*Lavandula vera, Lavandula officinalis*) is an-
    other of those plants so incredibly useful in cosmet-
    ics. Along with Rose and Comfrey, it could be all that
    one needs. The plant is low and shrubby and seems to
    grow anywhere, including wet and foggy San Fran-
    cisco. My plants produce three to four sets of flowers a
    year. Ideally, Lavender is grown in good loam over
    chalky well-drained soil in an open, dry, sunny posi-
    tion, free from dampness in the winter.

    The oil is distilled from the flower and leaf tops. It
    was used in earlier days as a condiment and to flavor
    dishes (it was said to comfort the stomach). It is now
    employed as an aromatic, carminative, and nervine.
    Lavender oil applied externally is used for stimulating
    sore, exhausted muscles and to rub on sprains, strains,

and stiff joints. It is also applied to a brush and brushed on the hair to stimulate hair growth; it works especially well mixed with oil of Basil, though oil of Rosemary is a considerably cheaper substitute. The oil and spirit are especially good when taken internally for all sorts of pains in the head and for the brain, as a restorative and tonic against faintness, weakness, giddiness, spasms, colic, vertigo—and with oil of Rosemary for loss of memory, it relieves melancholy and raises the spirits. Externally, a few drops in a hot footbath is used for fatigue, toothache, neuralgia, sprains, and rheumatism. A few drops of Lavender rubbed on the temples is very nice for a nervous headache.

A tea brewed from the tops is excellent to relieve a headache that results from fatigue and exhaustion or for stimulation when you need to wake up. For this purpose it is superb, especially when mixed with scented Geranium leaf, Rosemary, and Comfrey.

Fomentation of Lavender in bags can be used as an anesthetic to relieve pain or as an application or mask for the face.

A distilled water of Lavender and Licorice is used as a gargle for hoarseness and loss of voice. It is applied as an antiseptic for swabbing pimples, wounds, acne, or sores. The water is used as a wash for puffy eyes, bruises, bites, and other minor external sores or blemishes to normalize the sebaceous glands and reduce puffiness, and as a hair rinse to reduce oiliness.

The dried plant is added to baths and facial steaming herbs to stimulate the complexion, cleanse the skin, and act as an aromatic astringent; it can be mixed with Rosemary, Comfrey, and Rose. The dried plant is also one of the most commonly used plants in potpourris and sachets.

All in all, Lavender has an extensive cosmetic reputation in most types of lotions, potions, baths, after-shaves, waters, washes, soaps, etc.

Lemon (*Citrus limon, C. medica,* var. *limona*) is used extensively in perfumery and masculine cosmetics to provide that fresh scent that seems to be one of the most preferred. Lemon is an aromatic astringent and is used in many, many ways. The dried or fresh peel is added to bath herbs, facial steaming herbs, or to pot-pourris or herbal mixtures; used as a decoction for normal to oily hair or added directly to vinegar rinses for hair or face. Fresh Lemon juice can be applied directly to minor cuts or wounds, an excellent, albeit itchy, application to herpes and pruritis of the scrotum (also called hot itchy balls). Diluted Lemon juice makes an excellent final rinse for hair or face. A halved Lemon applied to horny elbows helps get rid of the scaly flesh; however, the inner rough side of the thick-skinned Avocado peel actually works better. Lemon juice rinse counteracts the alkalinity of shampoo and helps to get rid of dandruff. It is used as a gargle for sore throat, and as an application for sunburn. Suck on a Lemon to get rid of hiccups or for hysterical heartbeat. Add dried Lemon to sleep pillows, where it acts as a soothing refresher and, added to Rosemary, it helps people who sleep too heavily to wake up.

Lemongrass (*Cymbopogon citratus*) can be purchased from a few nurseries (try Hilltop Herb Farm—Texas). The plant is basically a tropical grass; however, I have had good results growing it here in San Francisco against a sunny wall and in a very deep pot. The grass is used in bath herbs, facial herbs, and hair rinse herbs. It is used to normalize overactive oil glands; as such it is useful for dry and oily skin, dandruff, and related skin problems. It is a source of commercial vitamin A. The oil is used in perfumery for inexpensive soaps and various other types of cosmetics.

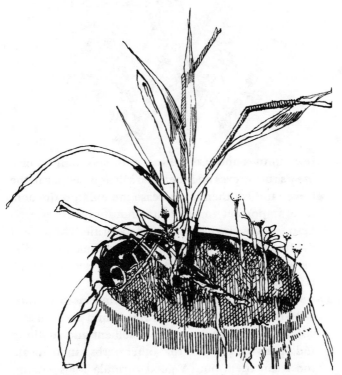

Lemon Verbena (*Lippia citriodora*) called Cédron in Mexico, when made into a tea, relieves indigestion and insomnia. The leaves are Lemon scented and used in bath herbs and facial herbs as a pore stimulant and in Lemon-scented potpourris. The oil produced by steam distillation is used in various cosmetics and in soapmaking.

Lettuce (*Lactuca sativa*—domestic; *L. virosa*—wild) leaves —wild and domestic—are used as a very effective wash for pimply skin or sore eyes. My Italian relatives suggest that a nursing mother simmer Lettuce for a

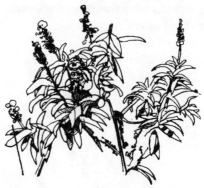

few minutes and use the water for sore nipples or a baby's runny eyes and then add salt and pepper to the leaves and eat them to increase the milk production. (It is important that you use nonsprayed Lettuce.) Lettuce tea is also used as a mild soporific. The juice of the fresh Lettuce is employed in soap-making and in the making of lotions and potions for sore or rough skin and to soothe a sunburn.

Licorice (*Glycyrrhiza glabra*) root is mainly used medicinally, but in cosmetics it has a unique and potent use in facial steaming herbs as it is emollient and soothing and opens the pores so that other herbs can medicate and clean them out. A good formula for steaming herbs is ⅓ Licorice root, ⅓ Comfrey root or leaf, and ⅓ medicating herbs such as Camomile or Lavender.

Lilac (*Syringa vulgaris*) flowers are occasionally dried and used in potpourris and sometimes infused in oil for the scent.

Lilies (*Lilium candidum*—Madonna Lily, used for burns and scars; *L. tigrinum*—used in Szechuan-style food, and in tincture to relieve morning sickness) have a long and interesting reputation as a cosmetic ingredient in all types of lotions, potions, and wrinkle creams. Most Lilies are soothing, emollient, and slightly astringent; they are often used for sore skin or for burns and scalds. Oils and ointments made from the dried bulbs are used for aching muscles and contracted or sore tendons.

🔥 **Lily of the Valley** (*Convallaria majalis*) flowers soaked in white wine are rubbed on the temples for a headache, drunk occasionally to strengthen the memory (they also act as a heart stimulant), and rubbed on aching joints to ease joint pain. The flowers are used in aromatherapy as a mild soporific; infused in oil, they make a unique and pleasant soothing massage oil.

🔥 **Lime** (*Citrus aurantifolia* or *C. limetta*) peel is used in potpourris, and Lime juice, as an astringent, is used in much the same way as Lemon juice. The juice diluted with water makes an effective mild skin freshener. The oil can be used as a scent for soaps, shampoos, and other cosmetic preparations, especially in masculine colognes and aftershave lotions.

Linden (*Tilia Europaea*) also known as Lime or Tilia, is commonly used as a sedative tea; however, when used in the bath it also acts as a mild sedative—both diaphoretic and antiseptic—for a hyperactive or hysterical person. The flowers are very cooling and relaxing when used internally or externally, and when infused in oil they give the same relaxing effect when massaged on the body.

Liverworts (*Anemone hepatica, Hepatica Americana*) are used as poultices or in bath herbs for mild disorders of the skin, including spots, freckles, and pimples.

🔥 **Lobelia** (*Lobelia inflata*) is occasionally used externally as a compress for skin irritations or breakouts.

🔥 **Logwood Chips** (*Haematoxylon campechianum*) are occasionally used as an antiseptic wash for sores of the skin where they act as an astringent.

Loosestrife (*Lythrum salicaria*), also called Purple Loosestrife, has been used as a wash for sore eyes, as a gargle for sore throat, and as a wash for sores. It acts as an astringent, demulcent, and emollient.

🕸 **Lotus** (*Nymphaea lutea, Zizyphus lotus*) root is used as a cleansing vaginal douche. The fragrant flowers are employed in perfumery or infused in oil and used for massage as a relaxant.

🕸 **Lovage** (*Levisticum officinale*) root in decoction is used as a face wash to remove freckles and spots and is very good in mixtures of bath herbs as an aromatic and mild diaphoretic.

Lupin flowers from the order *Leguminosae* are cleansing, cooling, and used in all types of lotions and potions on skin scabs and sores; they help scabby, dandruffy scalp and are used in soapmaking. Powdered Lupin seeds are dusted on blemishes to help heal them. (See also Bean Flowers.)

Luffa (*Luffa cylindrica, L. aegyptiaca*) is the fibrous skeleton of a gourd, and it is used as a stimulating, cleansing, scale-removing washcloth for the body. Excellent for underactive tissues. Now available at health food stores, fine department stores, and pharmacies. Also called Loofah.

🕸 **Mace** (*Myristica fragrans*) is the external covering of the Nutmeg and is used in perfumery and soapmaking. An ointment of Mace, Comfrey root, and Nutmeg is used as a counterirritant massage for arthritis and rheumatism.

🕸 **Madder** (*Rubia tinctorum*) as a dye is used in cosmetics to color the lips or cheeks.

🕸 **Magnolia** (*Magnolia spp.*) flowers are occasionally used in perfumery to yield an essential oil; however, they are not really exploited for the production of perfume oil. The scent is very soothing and exotic.

Maidenhair Fern See Ferns.

Mallow (any plant of the order *Malvaceae*) These plants are all used for their soothing emollient effects in creams, lotions, decoctions, and concoctions, and have many uses both medicinally and cosmetically. The roots and seeds boiled in white wine and massaged into the breasts ease swelling. The seeds can be steeped in vinegar and used as a skin wash, and the leaves bruised and laid on itchy insect bites to soothe them. Boil the juice in oil and smooth it over the skin for roughness or dry scabs; rub it into the scalp to keep the hair from falling out. (See also Marshmallow, Malva and Hollyhock.)

Malva rotundifolia also called Dwarf Mallow or Blue Malva, has pale purple flowers that are used in potpourris and, with the leaves, used in bath herbs for emolliency.

Malva sylvestris, called the Blue or Common Mallow (about 4 feet tall and bushy), has purple flowers used in potpourris; its leaves are employed in bath herbs and poultices as an emollient.

🕸 **Mandrake** (*Podophyllum peltatum*) The American kind is used in preparations to remove warts.

🕸 **Mangrove** (*Rhizophora mangle*) wood is hard and durable and its bark is very astringent. Occasionally it is applied as an astringent wash for skin blemishes. The fruit is said to be sweet and nourishing.

Maple (any tree of the order *Aceraceae, Acer campestre* —Common Maple; *A. saccharinum, A. rubrum*— Red Maple) bark is used much like Oak bark as it is astringent. Occasionally it is applied cosmetically.

Marigold (*Calendula officinalis,* and often *Tagetes spp.*) flowers are used in water infusions as a wash for sore, irritated skin or eyes and as a lightening rinse for the hair. It is a stimulant and diaphoretic and terrific in bath herbs or facial herb mixtures. For a little baby's bath, a mixture of Camomile, Marigold, and Comfrey is great as a skin soother; it is also useful as a wash for diaper rash and cradle cap. Powdered Marigold flowers, either by themselves or mixed half and half with powdered Camomile and talcum, make a wonderful body powder that is delicate enough for a newborn. A poultice of Marigold is good for sores or other external afflictions and is one of the few herbs recommended for varicose veins. Also, when infused in vinegar Marigolds become a facial wash and hair rinse.

Marjoram (*Origanum majorana*) The sweet type is powdered and used as a sneezing powder to clear the head and sinuses. It acts on the nervous system and is said to help overly erotic persons. It is a mild external antiseptic. The oil is used externally for headache, sprains, bruises, etc., and also as an emmenagogue. It is excellent in bath herb mixtures and is used to stimulate the sense of touch.

Marshmallow (*Althaea officinalis*) root is soothing, emollient, and contains much mucilage; its efficacy is increased when mixed with Comfrey root; and it is used with the leaves as a poultice for inflammations, bruises, strains, and sprains. It is generally applied medicinally, but is quite effective cosmetically in lotions and potions for sore skin or blemishes, as an eyewash, and in bath or facial herbs.

▨ **Mastic** (*Pistacia lentiscus*) is used occasionally as a chewing resin to improve the breath.

Meadowsweet (*Filipendula ulmaria, Spiraea ulmaria*) is an aromatic, diaphoretic, mild astringent and as such is used in bath herb mixtures and facial steaming mixtures. It aids in the cure of skin eruptions, and as an ingredient in massage oil helps rheumatism. Meadowsweet water as a wash is also used for skin blemishes.

Melilot (*Melilotus officinalis, M. alba, M. arvensis*), also called Hayflower, is used in an excellent hangover remedy as follows: 1 oz. Melilot and ½ oz. Sage infused in 1 cup white vinegar and 1 cup Rosewater for 1 week. Strain and use as a head wash or compress for head pains. Melilot has a similar smell to Tonka, new-mown Hay, and Woodruff (the smell is due to coumarin). Melilot plus Comfrey makes an excellent, relaxing, cleansing bath herb mixture. As a tea taken regularly, it acts as a natural deodorant. The herb also makes a good moth repellent either by itself or mixed with other herbs.

Melons of all types from the order *Cucurbitaceae* are much used in cosmetics as facial masks; the pulp mashed and added to Cornmeal, Oatmeal, or other types of meal such as Almond makes an excellent cleansing scrub. The Watermelon is good for normal to oily skin and the Casaba, Honeydew, and Cantaloupe are generally used for dry skin. Melon slices are also helpful as compresses for sore or tired eyes.

Milkweed See Asclepias.

Mimosa perfume from *Acacia decurrens* is an intensely fragrant oil that will generally act to round off the "rough notes from synthetic materials"—*Perfume and Flavor Materials of Natural Origin.* (See Acacia for uses of the flowers.)

Mints of all kinds are aromatic stimulants, somewhat astringent, which yield wonderfully fragrant oils by dis-

MINT

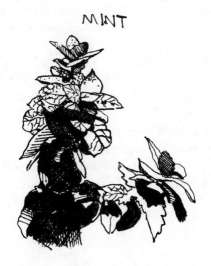

tillation: Applemint—*Mentha gentilis* (in England called Gingermint); Bergamot Mint or Orange Mint —*M. citrata;* Horsemint (American)—*Monarda punctata;* Horsemint (English)—*M. sylvestris;* Pennyroyal —*M. pulegium;* Peppermint—*M. piperita;* Pineapple Mint—*M. rotundifolia variegata;* Spearmint—*M. viridis;* Watermint—*M. aquatica.* There are many more Mints and hybrids but these are the usual cosmetic types. Spearmint is used in baths with Lemon balm and other herbs; it feels good and strengthens the nerves and muscles. The tea is used as a stomachic. Any of the Mints used in the bath will be stimulative and restorative; Mint inhaled as one would use smelling salts is a stimulant. In earlier times, Mint was used especially as a scent for the arms, with Rosemary as a tea, and inhaled to stimulate the memory. A poultice of Rose leaves and Spearmint is used on the head as a tranquilizer to help one to sleep. Mint with Rosemary and vinegar becomes a wash for dandruff. A strong infusion of Mint is used for chapped hands, especially when mixed with Almond meal. Spearmint is mostly used in cooking, while Peppermint is used in medicine and cosmetics. To tell the difference between the Spearmint and Peppermint, take a bit of both (oil or plant) in your mouth, then suck air in through pursed lips—Peppermint produces a hot aromatic taste at first, and afterward produces a sensation of cold in the mouth caused by the menthol it contains. About 300 pounds of the fresh plant will produce about 1 pound of the essential oil. All the Mints are terrific in bath herb mixtures as stimulating restoratives, as medication for the pores in facial herbs, as stimulating ingredients in facials, and as a component in soapmaking, mouthwash, lotions, potions, creams, mixed with honey, in hair rinse herbs, in massage oils for aching muscles, and as a compress for headache. Horsemint is especially good in shampoos and herb and vinegar rinses for dandruff. Pennyroyal is best in facial mixtures and as an insect repellent. Apple and Pineapple Mint are terrific in the bath and in potpourris. Spearmint is delicious as a tea, and Peppermint is great wherever its menthol content is needed in medicinal cosmetics. Indeed, Mint is one of the six best cosmetic herbs (Rose, Thyme, Comfrey, Mint, Lavender, Rosemary).

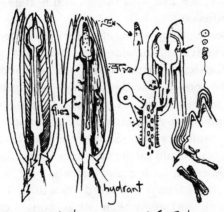

moonsocket or duck's left foot bush, constituent parts etc, and unrelated but hopefully perhaps nonetheless interesting details...

Morning Glory (*Iponaea spp.*, *Convolvulus spp.*) flowers are occasionally used as a compress for sore or tired eyes. They also can be used in herbal hair rinses to brighten hair.

Moss (*Lycopodium clavatum*—Common Club Moss; *Sphagnum cymbifolium*) has many and varied uses; most of them are medicinal but a few are cosmetic. Some of the Mosses, such as Common Club Moss, are dried and used as a body powder for chafing or itchy scratchy skin, or for skin diseases such as eczema. (See Irish Moss, which is actually not a moss but a seaplant.)

🜍 **Mugwort** (*Artemisia vulgaris*) is used in bath herb mixtures, especially with Camomile and Agrimony for sore, aching muscles or as a rub in a liniment or massage oil for overexertion. In aromatherapy inhaling the Mugwort is said to open the third eye, sleeping on it is supposed to reveal dreams of the future, and it is the herb used by the Chinese in moxas. (For clairvoyance, mix with Yarrow and Borage and take as an infusion.)

🜍 **Mulberry** (*Morus nigra, M. rubra*) dedicated to Minerva. The fruit of the oldest tree is the best and is used for diseases of the throat and windpipe and afflictions of the mouth. The dark juice is astringent and can be used in facial masks and packs. At the corner of Tenth and A in my hometown was a park and in the park was a Mulberry tree. Summer always became summer when I could eat the dark juicy fruits of the tree, which generally stained my clothes as I sat in the old tree's arms. I always wondered when the silk worms would come and weave their silk cocoons. I can remember the smell of the dust rising from the paths of the park and the secret feeling of walking along those dark overgrown passages to find the Mulberry tree that was the harbinger of summer.

Mullein, Great (*Verbascum thapsus*) leaves and flowers are used wherever astringent and emollient properties are needed. The yellow flowers are added to hair rinse mixtures for light to blond hair or to rinses for oily hair. A thick decoction of flowers makes a hair dye. The flowers steeped in olive oil are used as an application for sores or a massage oil for aching muscles.

Mustard seed (*Brassica alba*—mustard plaster, *B. nigra*—footbath) infusion in hot water is a footbath for sore, aching feet. Very stimulating. Mustard flowers in California are bright yellow and often grow in the fields alongside the Artichokes. These flowers can be used along with Camomile and Marigold as a stimulating wash.

Myrrh (*Commiphora myrrha, C. balsamodendroni*) is one of the oldest perfume materials known. It is traditionally used in cosmetics (though it is more medicinal than cosmetic), in mouthwashes, tooth powders, and toothpaste as an aromatic astringent. Smells nice too!

Myrtle (*Myrtus communis*) belongs to Venus and is thought to have been used by her as an intimate toilet water. The leaves can be used for various purposes: as an antiseptic, or a mild astringent in mixtures of herbs for vaginal douching. The leaves are very fragrant and are sometimes dried and used in linen closets to scent linen and towels; they are also an aromatic astringent in bath herbs. Myrtle oil is used in perfumery as a top note rather than as a fixative and blends with herbal oils such as Lavender, Rosemary, Clary, or Bergamot oil in colognes.

Narcissus (*Narcissus tazetta*) *A Modern Herbal* states that "the Arabians recommended the oil be used for curing baldness and as an aphrodisiac." (See also Daffodil and Jonquil.)

Nasturtium (*Tropaeolum majus*) flowers are used in bath herbs as an astringent and in hair rinses for dark blond to red hair; also delicious on salads.

Neroli oil is extracted from the flowers of the Bitter Orange and the Sweet Orange. When the extraction is from Bitter Orange flowers it is called Neroli Bigarde, and when from Sweet Orange it is called Neroli Portugal. This oil is used in perfumery and is highly valuable. It is used in aromatherapy for soothing the nerves, and in sleep pillows to help one fall asleep.

Nettles (*Urtica dioica*) are used mainly in herbal baths to stimulate the skin and to improve circulation (some-

times in wake-up baths or baths for arthritis). In herbal hair rinses, it stimulates growth and improves the
condition of the scalp. For shiny, glossy hair, make an
infusion of Nettle and Rosemary, brush into the hair,
and rub onto the scalp every day. It can also be infused
in vinegar instead of water, and used for the scalp.
Use only in the dried form. The young leaves contain
iron and are said to be good for the complexion as
they are a "blood purifier" and should be eaten often.
(See Chapter XX for Mike's Nettle Bath.)

Nutmeg (*Myristica fragrans*) extract is used in perfumery, especially in combination with such other
scents as Sandalwood, Lavender, Patchouli, and Vetivert, and in the spicy type of aftershave lotions and
other kinds of men's cosmetics. Nutmeg is used as a
massage oil to stimulate circulation and in all rheumatic pains and achey joints. It is used externally as a
gentle stimulant.

Oak (from many species of *Quercus*) bark is an antiseptic
astringent and is used wherever one is needed. It is
not terribly effective in cosmetics and has much
greater application as a medicinal. Mixed with other
herbs such as Mint and Comfrey, it makes a pleasant
wash for sore or skin eruptions, or as a mouthwash.
The Indians use the juice of the Valley Oak galls as an
eyewash.

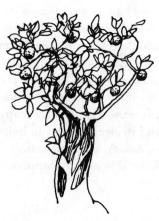

Oakmoss (*Evernia prunastri*) is a lichen, that is, it is formed from a fungus plus an alga. The resin from this lichen is one of the oldest botanical substances known to man and is used in perfumery and in soapmaking. Powdered Oakmoss is used as a basis for a body powder called Chypre. Rush baskets filled with Oakmoss have been found in the tombs of the Pharaohs of ancient Egypt. When fresh, it is scentless, but after it is dried and stored, it develops a musky Lavender-like scent. Used as a fixative in perfumery.

Oats and Oatmeal (*Avena sativa*) are among the most useful items on the home cosmetic shelf. Cook Oats and put the resultant gruel into a loose cheesecloth bag and add to the bath water to make a soothing liquid for itchy skin or when you have numerous insect bites. Oatmeal bath water is also good to soothe a baby's diaper rash or any type of body rash. Oats coarsely ground and mixed with honey make an excellent facial scrub. Oat flakes mixed with water, yogurt, milk, or any other liquid are excellent as a facial mask, especially after steaming the pores with herbs. Oatmeal, plus Almond meal and honey, is terrific to soften the skin; when rubbed into the hands it cleans, softens, and protects. Oatmeal can also be added to soaps for cleansing.

Oleander (*Nerium oleander*) is demulcent and emollient, and I have used this flower that smells rather like talcum powder as a scented addition to talc.

Olive oil (*Olea Europaea*) is an excellent all-purpose addition to cosmetics, massage and body oils, and lotions. I consider it the best oil for all these purposes. It makes an excellent soap, very hard and very mild on the skin. Add a little Lemon juice to Olive oil, and you can use it either as a soothing application to pruritis or as the beginnings of a delicious salad dressing. Instead of commercial baby oil, use Olive oil that has had

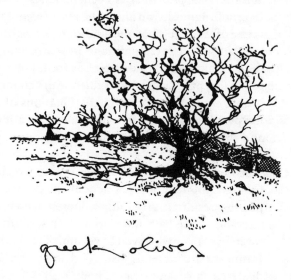

green olives

Camomile flowers infused in it; it is much better and more soothing for the baby's skin, and is also an application for cradle cap to facilitate the removal of the crusts. A mixture of Rosemary oil and Olive oil makes an excellent tonic for dry hair or as a hot oil massage for a sluggish scalp. Also used as a cuticle oil and foot massage, with coconut oil and vitamin E to erase stretch marks, and for pregnant stomachs and breasts so you won't get stretch marks. Also for insect bites, bruises, strains, sprains, and what have you.

Opopanax (*Opopanax spp.*) is used as a fixative in fragrant potpourris and as an ingredient in soapmaking.

Oranges (*Citrus vulgaris, C. aurantium,* var. *amara*—Bitter Orange; *C. sinensis, C. aurantium,* var. *dulcis*—Sweet Orange) have many uses. All parts can be used. The Sweet Orange peel is dried, cut, and added to bath herb mixtures as an antiseptic aromatic. Powdered, it can be mixed with any liquid and used as a facial mask for dry to oily skin. The Orange peel is a useful addition to herbal shampoos for oily scalp or dandruff, and it can also be infused in vinegar rinses for the same condition or in herbal rinses for light-colored or blond hair. Oil of Orange peel is used in perfumery, for flavors, or to scent various types of cosmetic preparations including creams and shampoos.

Orange flowers are best used in potpourris as their delicious scent is lost when they are cooked into lotions; they can be used in cold infusions of massage oils where the scent is very light and very soothing. Fresh Orange flowers can be macerated in oils or saturated fats to make cold creams and body creams. Orange flowers (bitter) yield Neroli oil by distillation and Orange flower absolute by extraction. The scent is very different for each, and I prefer the Orange flower absolute as it more resembles the pure fresh Orange flower. The concrete is very dark, brownish, and soft; the smell reminds me of days long past when I lived in the middle of an Orange grove and on certain delicious evenings went to sleep and then woke up to this strong, deeply sweet scent. The blossoms are added to facial herbs as a hydrating agent and in face packs for young-looking skin.

Bitter Orange peel is used in bath herb mixtures for its particular astringency, and oil of Bitter Orange is generally used in liqueurs such as triple sec and also for soft drinks.

Orange leaf and twigs are used in aromatherapy for their seeming ability to sharpen awareness. The oil is called Petitgrain and is used in soapmaking and in perfumery for its refreshing qualities.

The small immature fruits of the Orange tree are added to liqueurs such as curacao; I use them in my drawers for scenting, especially mixed up with the linen or lingerie.

Orange flower water is used in cooking or in lotions and facial rinses as a hydrating agent; it is a popular household cosmetic agent, but unfortunately does not keep very well and gets rancid and moldy and mildews easily.

Orchids See Vanilla.

Oregano (*Origanum vulgare*) is useful in bath herbs where it functions as a very mild painkiller (say for aching muscles), or in external poultices for aching muscles or feet. However, if Oregano is all that you have, and you are where the water is hard or drying, by all means use it as an afterbath or shower rinse to allay the bad effects of city water. Oil of Oregano is useful mixed with Olive oil and oil of Rosemary as a daily rub for an itchy scalp.

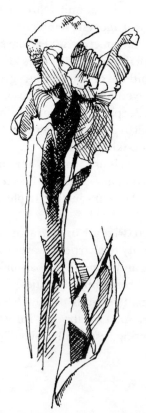

🔥 **Orris** (*Iris germanica, I. florentina, I. pallida*) root is the dried rhizome of the Florentine Iris. It has a very distinctive scent that can be likened to the aroma of Violets and is in fact used in Violet-scented body powder. The plant is available at several nurseries and Hemlock Hill Herb Farm in Litchfield, Connecticut. Orris root has fixative qualities in both potpourris and perfumery; it is a common ingredient in soapmaking and in fine cosmetics such as face powders and toilet water to remove freckles and spots. Powdered Orris is used in tooth powders, in the last rinse water of fine lingerie, in sachets, or body powder mixtures (however, it sometimes causes allergic reactions). The larger pieces are used in shampoos with other herbs, especially in shampoos for light hair or for scalp conditions. Whole pieces of the root are used as infant's teething rings.

Palmarosa (*Cymbopogon martini*, var. *motia*) oil is a substitute for pure Geranium oil (geraniol), and is used in perfumery and soapmaking.

Pandanus (*Pandanus odoratissimus*) flowers are steam distilled for the fragrant oil that is used in perfumery and soapmaking. The flowers can also be distilled in the home, and the resulting flower water used as a cosmetic wash such as Rosewater. The pollen of the Hawaiian Pandanus tree (the Hala or Lauhala) was at one time collected and used as an aphrodisiac.

🔥 **Pansy** (*Viola tricolor*), also called Heartsease, is extremely useful for the skin. It contains salicylic acid and is, therefore, an effective medicinal astringent in facial herbs, herbal rinses for the hair, bath herbs, lotions, creams, ointments, and especially as external fomentations for eczema and other skin diseases. It is especially nice for all types of skin disease in babies, such as cradle cap. Use the fresh leaves for pimples. It is cooling, emollient, and allays inflammation.

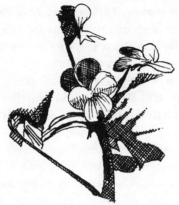

🌿 **Papayas** (*Carica papaya*) are one of the most effective plants for cosmetic problems. The ripe fruit is mashed and used in masks to degrease an oily complexion. The seeds can be mashed and mixed with Oatmeal as cleansing grains. The "milk" from the stalk is used as an exfoliant, but should be diluted. The leaf, dried and mixed with Cornmeal, is terrific as a mask for normal to oily skin and to remove scaly, crusty skin. The leaves, when fresh and mixed with Comfrey leaves, are used as an exfoliant. The Papaya is an effective aid to protein digestion, and the juice can be applied for a moment or two to exfoliate the upper lip area.

Paprika (*Capsicum spp.*) can be used in hair rinses for a reddish tinge or, when mixed with Henna as a dye, for a reddish-bronze color.

Parsley (*Petroselinum sativum*) when eaten daily, is said to be the key to good health and a clear complexion. It is a useful, cleansing, and medicating addition to all types of lotions and cosmetics for many skin problems including eczema and psoriasis. It is also useful in massage oils for the beneficial effects it produces on the skin. Parsley seed oil is used for special effects in perfumery.

🔥 **Passionflower** (*Passiflora incarnata*—herb; *P. edulis*—fruit) herb is used for its quieting, soothing effect in teas and bath herb mixtures. The flower is used in massage oils; the perfume oil is extracted by the enfleurage method. The Lilikoi (Passionflower fruit) is mashed and used in masks for cleansing.

Patchouli (*Pogostemon cablin, P. patchouli*) oil is produced by steam distillation. This is one of the most important perfumery plants and is used as a main scent, fixative, and blender. It is frequently used in soapmaking. The herb is also effective in trunks and drawers as a bug repellent; in aromatherapy and sleep pillows as a stimulant for those who can't wake up in the morning; in herbal bath mixtures with Comfrey and Ginseng to rejuvenate the skin; in potpourris with Rose, Vetivert, and Sandalwood. Powdered Patchouli and powdered Lemon peel make an effective underarm deodorant but have the disadvantage of staining light-colored clothes. In days past Indian shawls were authenticated by the smell of the Patchouli they were wrapped in for shipping.

🔥 **Pawale** (*Rumex giganteus*—Hawaiian Dock) bark or root is used in Hawaii as a decoction for skin diseases.

Peach (*Prunus persica*) blossoms are distilled to furnish a delicious liquor. Peach blossom syrup is a tonic for the system and acts as a mild laxative for children. Grieve says, "In America, the Peach is chiefly used for feeding pigs, and for making Peach Brandy"—an interesting observation. Peach leaves are used in facial masks and bath herbs as emollients, especially for normal to dry skin. Peach kernels are eaten (see Almond kernels), but can be dangerous to one's health. Peach kernel oil is used in fine cosmetics and soapmaking and in the making of fine hand lotions and massage and body oils. Peach kernels cooked in Apple cider vinegar are said to be a hair growth stimulator when rubbed daily onto the scalp. Fresh Peach flesh is an excellent poultice for irritated skin.

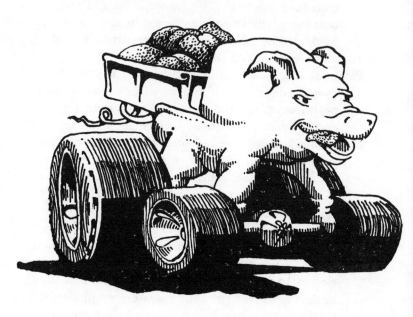

Pears (*Pyrus communis*) are mildly laxative and, if used externally, are soothing and cooling, especially for sore skin or sunburn. A slice of Pear laid across sore, tired eyes is very helpful. Pears can also be used in facial masks for normal to dry skin.

Peas (*Pisum sativum*) contain vitamin E and, when cooked, mashed, and applied to bruises and sores, act as a facial mask. Peas are a mild food useful for delicate digestions. They are used internally and externally for piles and varicose veins. The water the Peas are cooked in is good as a facial wash for all complexions.

Pelargonium See Geranium.

🔥 **Pennyroyal** (*Mentha pulegium*—European Pennyroyal; *Hedeoma pulegioides*—American Pennyroyal) is great in bath herbs as a diaphoretic to soothe burning or itching skin. A decoction of Pennyroyal rubbed on the body is a useful deodorant and insect repellant. The oil is employed in perfumery, especially for industrial uses. Yerba Buena is often mistakenly called American Pennyroyal (see also Mint).

ⓒ **Peony** (*Paeonia officinalis*) decoction is used for skin affections and pains in the extremities. As an external soak for the extremities, add Comfrey.

Pepper (*Piper nigrum*) grain decoction is used as a wash for *Tinea capitatis* (a fungus infection of the scalp).

Peppermint (*Mentha piperita*) Peppermint herb is used for its cooling and antiseptic effect in bath and facial herbs. The oil, which contains menthol, is an ingredient in many cosmetics, lipsticks, face creams, lotions, shaving creams, hair lotions, etc. The oil has a drying effect on the skin and hair, while the herb has an emollient effect. (See also Mint.)

ⓒ **Periwinkles** (*Vinca major, V. minor*) are used as astringent washes for all sorts of skin afflictions and in bath herb mixtures. Soothing and very healing. Fresh leaves can be used as a wash for cradle cap.

Peru, Balsam See Balsam of Peru.

ⓒ **Peruvian** (*Cinchona spp.*) bark is used in the making of tooth powders for its cleansing astringency.

ⓒ **Petitgrain** oil is steam distilled from the leaves and twigs of the Bitter Orange tree. In aromatherapy the scent is inhaled to sharpen awareness. The oil is also used in soapmaking, lotions, and other cosmetics such as aftershave lotion.

Pikake (*Jasminum sambac*) See Jasmine.

Pimpernel, Scarlet (*Anagallis arvensis*) has an old reputation as a cosmetic herb, used as a wash for general complexion care, pimples, and freckles. It is slightly astringent and diaphoretic. It is a specific for the liver.

Pine (of many species) produces many useful products such as room deodorants; air fresheners; bath oils;

turpentine, which is produced by distillation and applied as an external rub for aching joints, rheumatic and arthritic pains; and tar (impure turpentine). This tar is used extensively in dermatology for the manufacture of soaps and lotions to treat eczema, psoriasis, and other skin afflictions. Tar is stimulating and antiseptic. Pine needles are used extensively in bath herb mixtures for stimulating and soothing for skin. Terrific as a wake-up bath or shower in the morning. Pine needles make a delightful aromatic "Sleep and Dream Pillow," available from New Age Creations, S.F.

Pineapple (*Ananas comosus, A. sativus*) juice and flesh are effective as an astringent wash for oily skin, as a mild exfoliating scrub, and is sipped or eaten frequently for sore throat.

Plantain (*Plantago major*) decoction is a stimulating, cleansing wash for sore, inflamed skin. It is also one of our favorite medicinal herbs, having many applications, although it sometimes blisters the skin and causes allergic reactions (see *Herbs & Things*). The American Indians called it white man's footsteps.

Plumeria (*Plumeria acuminata*—Melia; *P. rubra*—has more fragrance at night) also called Frangipani, is thought to have been used by the Aztecs—known as Cocaloxochite—as a powerful potion against fear and faintheartedness. The Plumeria is not utilized for perfume manufacture anywhere in the world, except by those few who make perfume oil at home; it has an absolutely delicious, delightful scent and makes me think of small, warm beaches, warm sun, and clear water. The flowers can be infused in oil or unscented creams for a pleasing massage or body cream.

Pomegranate (*Punica granatum*) juice makes an excellent external astringent for oily skin and, if any drips into your mouth, drink up for it is beneficial in relieving diarrhea. Can also be used as a body dye. Along

DWARF POMEGRANATE

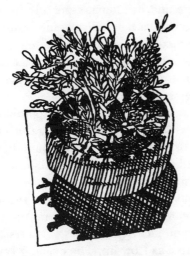

with Licorice, Camomile, and Henna, it is mentioned
in the Ebers Papyrus as an Egyptian herb.

Poppy, California (*Eschscholtzia californica*) was the *Copa
de Oro* or Cup of Gold of the Spaniards. These flowers
were eaten to relieve anxiety. The Placer County In-

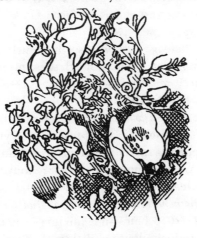

POPPY'S WORLD

dians boiled the greens like spinach and ate them. A tea or tincture of the whole plant was used as medicine for headache and insomnia, especially for children, and was said to be a nonaddictive substitute for morphine. The Spaniards would fry the entire plant in Olive oil, add scent, and use the resulting mixture as a super-stimulating hair oil said to promote growth and make hair glossy.

Potato (*Solanum tuberosum*) grated raw, placed on black and blue marks with an added bandage, will get rid of those discolorations within a few hours. Raw Potato juice is excellent to get rid of the itch and scratch of poison oak and also as an external application for any itchy skin. It's the potassium that does the job.

Primrose (*Primula vulgaris*) decoction makes an excellent astringent face wash. These flowers are used much the same as Cowslip. The evening Primrose is very fragrant, astringent, and sedative and is effective in bath herb mixtures. Some Primrose species cause irritation of the skin.

Prunes (*Prunus domestica*) are occasionally mashed and used by themselves—or mixed with Oatmeal—as a nourishing and cleansing facial mask. (See Monster Mask in Chapter IX.)

Psyllium (*Plantago psyllium*) seeds, which are soothing and emollient, are used much the same as Flax seeds.

Pyrethrum (*P. tanacetum*—Costmary; *P. carneum*—Persian Insect Powder; *P. cinerariefolium*—Dalmation Insect Powder; *P. parthenium*—Feverfew or Febriguge plant; *P. roseum*—Insect plant) Most of the Pyrethrums can be applied as insect repellents by making a water decoction and dabbing it on your body. The flowers make cleansing rinses for the scalp.

Quassia (*Picraena (Picrasma) excelsa, Quassia amara*) chips are added to hair rinse mixtures for cleansing the scalp and eliminating dandruff. Because they are light-colored wood, they are especially effective on light-colored hair.

🝠 **Quince** (*Pyrus cydonia, Cydonia oblonga*) is a plant sacred to Venus and is used to ward off the influence of the evil eye. The seeds, soaked in water, make a soothing emollient gel that is an excellent base for lotions and creams. The gel made with Rosewater or Witch Hazel water is a powerful nonalcoholic aftershave, nonstinging and very healing. Quince seeds can also be used in much the same manner as Flax seeds.

🝠**Ragweed** (*Ambrosia spp.*) also known as Ragwort, is occasionally used in herbal hair rinses as an astringent and antiseptic and to stimulate growth.

🝠 **Ragwort,** also known as Ragweed, should not be confused with real Ragweed. The Ragworts are *Senecio spp.* The common Ragwort, *S. vulgaris* (sometimes called common Groundsel), is a diaphoretic when added to the bath, and is a soothing ingredient in lotions for chapped hands with Flax gel and Arnica. *S. jacobaea,* or Ragwort, also known as St. Jameswort, is a cooling emollient astringent; its action is emphasized when combined with Comfrey root. It is an effective wash for the scalp or skin, for sores, and inflamed surfaces. (See also Groundsel.)

Raspberry (*Rubus idaeus*) leaf[1] contains a substance called fragarine, which seems to relax the muscles of the uterus and intestine and is, therefore, an excellent tea taken before and during childbirth. It is also a stimulating astringent in herbal hair rinses and bath herb mixtures, and, along with Comfrey and Licorice, it makes an excellent herb for facial packs and steams for oily skin.

Reindeer Moss, a species of *Cladonia,* is a pleasantly

---

[1] I have used it extensively and will have more to say in my forthcoming book, *The Herbal Mother and Child Book.*

scented lichen which when powdered is used as a substitute for Oakmoss in cosmetic powders.

Rice (*Oryza sativa*), white and powdered, makes an excellent nonirritating skin powder. Ricewater makes a soothing application for sunburn or sore skin; it is also effective in baths for infants, children, or adults to soothe irritated, sunburned, or windburned skin.

Rock Rose (*Cistus ladaniferus*) yields a resin, Labdanum, which is used extensively in soapmaking and in perfumery as a fixative and blender for its rich sweetness. Decoction of American Rock Rose is used to treat skin diseases as a wash.

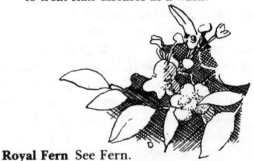

Royal Fern See Fern.

Roses are a group of shrubs found in the temperate areas of the world. The birthplace of the cultivated Rose is probably ancient Persia, where the oldest Rose was most likely a deep red color which suggested the myth of the Rose springing from the blood of Adonis. Otto of Rose was first extracted in 1612. Indeed, Roses were used since Roman times to float in wine; brides and bridegrooms were crowned with Roses; they were scattered at feasts and in the paths of the winners of games and contests, and worn as wreaths at feasts, especially as a preventative against drunkenness. The Rose was a sign of pleasure and a companion fit for wine. It was once the custom to suspend a Rose over the dinner table as a sign that all private conversations were to be held sacred (that is, sub rosa). The discovery of Otto of Rose by the Persians is very interesting:

According to a discourse on Roses written in 1844, a princess and her emperor, upon the celebration of their marriage in 1612, spent huge sums for an extravagant and luxurious party. They filled the canal that flowed through the flower gardens of the palace with Rosewater, and while walking along the bank of the canal, they noticed that an oily layer had collected on the surface. This layer was collected and immediately determined to have the most delicate of odors; it has since been termed Otto of Rose or Rose attar.

Two acres of Roses yield 10,000 pounds of Roses which, in turn, yield 1 pound of oil. This, in fact,

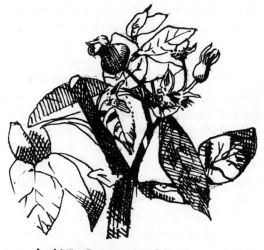

WILD ROSE HIPS

means that it takes approximately 30 Roses to make 1 drop of oil. There are many uses for Rosewater, Rose oil, and Rose petals in cosmetics, and you will find frequent mention of these products throughout Parts II, III, and IV of this book. Rose oil from the *Rosa centifolia* is called Rose de mai absolute and is processed in Morocco and France. It is used in perfumes, cosmetics, cold cream, and face powder perfumes. Otto of Rose is the essential oil obtained by steam distillation from the flowers of the Damask Rose in Bulgaria (*Rosa damascena,* also called the Bulgarian Rose). *Rose gallica,* the Apothecary Rose, was the traditional Rose of pharmacy (Provence Rose).

Briefly, Rosewater is an astringent tonic for the flesh; Rose oil is soothing both physically and emotionally; Rose petals are astringent and cleansing; and Rose vinegar is a soothing deodorant wash for the armpits and groin.

Rosemary (*Rosmarinus officinalis*) is another one of those plants having myriad applications in cosmetics. It has a fascinating history, being an herb of remembrance and therefore used both as a good luck herb for marriages and as a remembrance of death. The herb is used in baths as a diaphoretic and an astringent healer; it is also used in facial herbs; a decoction with Comfrey is good for all sorts of bruises and sores; a poultice with Camomile is good for pimples; an infusion with Nettle is excellent as a conditioner for the hair, especially dark hair; infused in oil, Rosemary is terrific for aching muscles; and infused in Olive oil with some essential oil of Rosemary, it is said to condition the scalp and stimulate hair growth. Pure essential oil of Rosemary makes an excellent hair conditioner (however, I prefer the more expensive oils of Lavender and Basil). A wonderfully fragrant hair conditioner can be made with 1 oz. of oil of Rosemary mixed with ½ oz. oil of Basil and ½ oz. oil of Lavender: A few drops brushed into the hair every day will condition and gloss it. Rosemary with Lavender is an excellent herbal stimulant tea if you are allergic to caffeine. And Rosemary oil is used in perfumery for colognes, waters, room deodorants, household sprays, disinfectants, insecticides, and soapmaking.

Safflower (*Carthamus tinctorius*) Also called Dyers Saffron. The oil is one of the most useful oils in cosmetics, being a base for many lotions and massage oils. The flowers are utilized in decoctions as a poultice for skin eruptions, pimples, and skin complaints.

Saffron Crocus (*Crocus sativus*) flowers in the fall and is usually cultivated for its bright yellow stigmas which are used primarily in cooking. It is used as a diaphoretic and an anodyne, as a water-soluble red dye in cosmetics and hair rinses, and in salves and lotions. However, since it is so expensive it has very limited cosmetic applicability. It grows in my garden, putting up its green shoots in the spring regularly but never flowering in the fall. This is probably due to the fact that it was not planted in the hottest part of the garden; it really needs lots of sun and heat to flower.

Sage oil in commerce is steam distilled from the Clary Sage (*Salvia sclarea*), Dalmatian Sage (*S. officinalis*), and Spanish Sage (*S. lavandulaefolia*). Sage oil is used in soap perfumery, in herb colognes as a blender, in industrial perfumes, and at home—straight or mixed with such oils as Lavender, Rosemary, and Basil

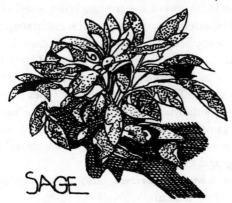

SAGE

—as a hair conditioner. (It is interesting to note that the Dalmatian Sage contains a substance called Thujone, also present in Wormwood, that part of absinthe that made it illegal in most of the world for being toxic and harmful to humans.) Dalmatian Sage also has excellent bactericidal value, although it can cause skin irritation, and is still used as a mouthwash and gargle. You can make a water infusion of Sage and Alum root for canker sores and a mouth cleanser. Goats Rue and Sage herb infusion will greatly ease aching muscles and sore, tired feet. Sage decoction drunk as a tea *and* applied as a hair rinse will darken the hair. Sage infusion or Sage as a facial wash will help to heal skin eruptions. Sage is terrific in an herbal bath, helps to check perspiration, and stimulates the skin.

Sagebrush (*Artemesia tridentata*) decoction can be drunk or eaten. Bathed in, it acts as a natural deodorant.

St. Johnswort (*Hypericum perforatum*) infused in oil makes a good massage oil for sore muscles. It is an aromatic astringent and mixed with shampoo herbs it cleanses the scalp.

Sandalwood (*Santalum album*) is one of the oldest known perfume materials; in fact, it has been used for over 4000 uninterrupted years. The oil is steam distilled from the wood of the tree and then used as a fixative and blender in perfumery and scent in soapmaking. It is also applied as an external disinfectant and antiseptic for sores and wounds. A personal friend has used this oil as an application for staph sores and feels that is is more efficacious than other types of medicines. The Sandalwood chips themselves are nice in bath herb mixtures as antiseptics, and the scent is thought to be rejuvenative, especially when mixed with Ginseng and Comfrey root.

Santolina Chaemycyparissus, also called Lavender Cotton, is used as an Arabian eyewash.

Sarsaparilla (*Smilax spp.*) is effective in bath herb mixtures as a cleansing diaphoretic, for soothing aching muscles, and as a wash for skin diseases. American Indians applied a decoction of the root on sore eyes.

🔥 **Sassafras** (*Sassafras albidum, S. officinale*) tea is a stimulating diaphoretic aromatic used as a wash for skin eruptions; mixed with Rosewater, it is useful as an eye-clearing wash; mixed with lanolin, it makes a good salve for skin diseases. A decoction of the bark is used to ease the itch of poison oak or as a mouthwash.

Savory Summer Savory (*Satureia hortensis*) is an annual, and Winter Savory (*S. montana*) is a perennial). I have both in my garden and use them mainly for culinary purposes and as an external application for insect bites. If you get a bee sting, quickly pick some Summer Savory and rub it vigorously on the affected area; it works almost instantly. Savory can also be mixed with Lavender and Rosemary for a very stimulating wake-up bath or tea.

Scotch Broom (*Cytisus scoparius*) flowers are used in hair rinse herbs as a yellow dye. (See also Broom.)

Seaweed has many cosmetic applications: Agar-agar is a vegetable gelatin which is a product of red algae used to make jellies and for stiffening silks. Carageenans, found in red algae, are used as a soothing demulcent or emollient and as an emulsifying agent in cosmetics. *Algin*, as sodium alginate, effectively reduces strontium uptake in the body; it is also used to thicken and stabilize soups, mayonnaise, and cosmetic lotions. Algin is found in brown Seaweeds, and as an emulsifier, it binds oily and watery fluids. Its chief commercial cosmetic use is in make-up.

The Chinese use Seaweed for abscesses; people of the South Seas use it for skin diseases and inflammations. Hawaiians eat the Limu to decrease fat and, indeed, this may be responsible for their low incidence of coronary occlusions. Seaweed, Kelp, and Dulse, powdered and mixed with baking soda and salt, are a wonderful addition to a bath to soothe aching or sunburned flesh.

Sedem (*Sedum spp.*), also called Stonecrop, is used as an astringent in any type of skin ointment and also as an ingredient in bath herbs.

Sesame (*Sesamum indicum*) oil is useful in all external applications: massage oil, bath oil, lotions, salves, creams, etc. It is a semidrying oil and best used in cosmetics for oily skin.

Slippery Elm See Elm, Slippery.

Snapdragons (*Antirrhinum majus*) are powerful antidotes to witchcraft. Combined with lanolin or oil, they make a useful salve for piles, bruises, or sores. A water decoction of the flowers is applied to soothe irritated skin. The tea is said to improve the sense of taste.

Soap Bark (*Quillaja saponaria*) mixed with water forms a detergent (cleansing) lather, which relieves itchy scalp or dandruff; this can also act as a wash for skin eruptions or skin sores, itchy feet, or athlete's foot. It can also be used for washing the hair and delicate clothing items such as baby clothes or fine woolens.

Soapwort (*Saponaria officinalis*) Used same as above. Has also been used to restore luster to ancient woolens that have been stored for some time.

Solomon's Seal (*Polygonatum multiflorum*) decoction is used as a wash for pimples, freckles, other spots, sores, bruises, and as an ingredient in herbal creams. The powdered root cooked in lanolin or oil and applied as a poultice is used to relieve a black eye.

Sorrel (both the Wood Oxalis, *Oxalis acetosella*, and the French Sorrel, *Rumex scutatus*) is used as an antiseptic wash for the skin and for any type of skin eruption.

Southernwood (*Artemisia abrotanum*) decoction boiled with Barley is applied as a wash for pimples and sores;

a mixture of the ashes infused in Olive oil and rubbed into the scalp daily is said to be a growth stimulant; fresh Southernwood mixed with Lemon balm and inhaled is said to keep you from being drowsy in boring classrooms; it is also used as a growth stimulant with Rosemary and Nettle in herbal shampoos and hair rinse mixtures.

⚘ **Sow Thistle** (*Sonchus oleraceus*—common type; *S. arvensis* Corn Thistle; *S. alpinus*—Mountain Thistle) juice is used as an external application to cleanse the face and make it shiny.

Soy (*Glycine soja*) oil is used in all types of cosmetic preparations, as a base in massage and body oils.

Spearmint See Mint.

Speedwell (*Veronica officinalis*—common; *V. chamaedrys* —Germander Speedwell) is used as an astringent, and by water infusion, it is used as a cosmetic wash for skin complaints and diseases such as eczema or psoriasis.

⚘ **Spruce Needles.** Spruce oil from *Tsuga canadensis* is pleasant in the bath and is used commercially in soapmaking, room deodorants, bath preparations, and many other types of household products. (See also Pine Needles.)

Storax is usually called Styrax in perfumery; this is the deliciously scented natural Balsam formed as a pathological product of the *Liquidambar orientalis*, a tree native to Asia Minor. American Styrax is produced from the *L. styraciflua*. The essential oil is steam distilled from the crude Styrax, is soluble in alcohol, and is used in perfumery. Mixed with Olive oil, it is a treatment for scabies and other external skin afflictions. It is used in soapmaking. The ground resin is used in potpourris and sachets.

⚘ **Strawberry** (*Frageria vesca* and other spp.) leaves make a useful astringent herb in bath herb or facial herb

mixes; they are especially useful for oily skin. The ripe
fruits mashed and applied as a pack either alone or
with Oatmeal or other meal are effective in cleansing
an oily complexion. The juice of the fruit or leaf can
be added to lotions or creams.

🔥 **Sumbul** (*Ferula sumbul*) root is used in perfumery and
cosmetics as a scent and fixative of great virtue. The
oil is obtained by steam distillation (also called Musk
root).

Sunflower (*Helianthus annuus*) seeds make an excellent
nutritious food, both internally—for the body—and
externally—for the skin. Grind them up and mix with
a liquid (milk for dry skin and yogurt for oily skin) to
form a paste, apply to a clean, damp face, let dry, and
then rinse off with warm water. Sunflower oil is especially useful for oily skin. The yellow Sunflower petals
are used as an ingredient in herbal hair rinses, especially for blond or light-colored hair.

Sweet Pea (*Lathyrus latifolius*) flower oil can be obtained at
home by the enfleurage method and used in bath or
massage oils. There has been some commercial use of
Sweet Pea in the perfume industry of Bermuda.

Tagetes (*Tagetes patula*). The essential oil is used rather
like the European Calendula. The Aztecs called it
Iyauhtli (Cloud Plant) and drank the delicious
Tarragon-scented tea. They also used the reddish-
gold flowers as a rinse for the hair. Also called Pericon
in Mexico. (See also Marigold.)

🔥 **Tangerine** (*Citrus reticulata*) peels, powdered and ground,
can be combined with Cornmeal and used as effective
beauty washing grains or mixed with yogurt as a face
pack. It is especially effective on oily or pimply complexions as it contains a fair quantity of vitamin A (420
I.U./100 gr.). The juice can be used as a complexion
rinse or wash in much the same manner as Lemon
juice or Orange juice. Tangerine oil is machine

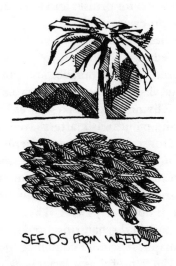

SEEDS FROM WEEDS

pressed and is employed in perfumery as a cologne modifier.

Tansy (*Tanacetum vulgare*) flowers have been used for herbal cosmetics for hundreds of years; mixed with Camomile flowers, Strawberry leaves, Comfrey root, and distilled in milk or Rosewater, this makes an excellent and soothing complexion cleanser for everyone. Tansy lotions are especially effective on blemishes or pimples. Tansy oil is steam distilled but has little applicability in perfumery.

Tapioca (*Manihot esculenta, M. utilissima*), also called Manioc or Cassava, cooked with milk makes a soothing application to tired, windburned skin.

Tartaric acid, available at pharmacies, is used in fizzy types of bath salts and cosmetics.

Tea (*Thea sinensis, Camellia thea*) The common tea bag makes an effective, stimulating astringent wash for the skin, for sunburn, as a poultice for baggy eyes, or a compress for a headache or tired eyes.

Teazles (*Dipsacus sylvestris*—common Teazle) are used as an application for bruises and warts and as a cosmetic water or an eyewash.

⚜ **Theobroma** See Cacao.

Thuja See Cedar.

Thyme is used as an aromatic, antiseptic, diaphoretic, stimulant, disinfectant, and is very useful in cosmetic lotions. Thyme water makes an effective underarm deodorant, mouthwash, aftershave lotion, and external wash for scabies. Thyme (antiseptic) with Comfrey (emollient), Lavender (astringent), and Mint (aromatic) makes a terrific bath herb mixture that will smooth and soothe the skin. Men, especially, like this combination as it is not overly sweet. Thyme is effective in all types of bath herbs, hair rinse, and shampoos. It is also a mild diaphoretic, and combined with Licorice and Comfrey, it is useful as a facial pack or herbal steam for psoriasis, eczema, and other types of skin problems. Oil of Thyme is used to scent all types of men's and women's cosmetics, in soapmaking, and in perfumery. Thyme oil is produced from *Thymus vulgaris;* Origanum oil from *T. capitatus* or *Origanum vulgare;* Wild Marjoram oil from *T. masticina* or *O. vulgare;* Sweet Marjoram oil from *Majorana hortensis.*

Tilia See Linden.

⚜ **Tobacco** (*Nicotiana tabacum*) leaf absolute yields a substance called Tabac that is employed in soapmaking and for masculine or dry effects in perfumery. The leaves are not used in cosmetics because the nicotine is very poisonous and readily absorbed by the skin.

⚜ **Tragacanth** (*Astralagus gummifer*), an emollient and demulcent, yields a thick mucilage; combined with water, it is very useful in vegetable cosmetics for lotions and creams.

⚜ **Tuberose** (*Polyanthes tuberosa*) flowers yield a wonderfully fragrant oil by enfleurage that is very effective in massage and body oils. During May, June, and

July, when my plants bloom, I drop these delicious-smelling flowers into champagne or white wine. The wine takes on the flowers' scent and is said by some to be wildly erotic. This is one of those flowers that produce and exhale their oil long after being picked. The scent is inhaled to enhance all the senses. In commercial perfumery, the blossoms are picked just before they open and the oil extracted by enfleurage.

Vanilla (*Vanilla planifolia, V. aromatica*) beans are used in dry potpourris, in hot chocolate as an aphrodisiac, and infused in oils as a body or massage oil. The Vanilla bean is commercially extracted to yield Vanilla extracts that are used in flavors, baking, chocolate making, soft drinks, pharmaceutical products, liqueurs, candies, etc., as well as perfumery and soapmaking.

Verbena, Lemon See Lemon Verbena.

Vetivert (*Vetiveria zizanioides, Andropogon zizanioides*) root is used in bath herb mixtures to cleanse and soothe the skin. It works especially well with herbs such as Patchouli, Sandalwood, and Comfrey. It is added to potpourris as a fixative. The oil is obtained by steam distillation and used in soapmaking and perfumery.

Violet, Sweet (*Viola odorata*) is one of the herbs mentioned in ancient Greek history. We use Sweet Violets, leaf and flower, fresh and dried, in teas and baths for their soothing and slight astringent abilities; they contain salicylic acid and are extremely high in vitamins A and C. Thus they make very useful facial waters for all skin afflictions or for just plain normal skin. Violet water is a wonderful aftershave or wash for a baby's skin. The leaves and flowers, simmered in oil, with lanolin or beeswax added, make excellent cold creams or lotions for daily use. Violet flower oil is hardly ever made as it is incredibly expensive (most Violet perfume is synthetic), but it can be made at home by the enfleurage method, and massage or body oils can be made by cold infusion of the flower. (See also Pansy, *V. tricolor*.)

Wallflower (*Cheiranthus cheiri*) oil can be made at home by the enfleurage method, diluted with Almond oil, and used as massage to soothe the nerves. Indeed, this plant has been known in the eastern Mediterranean for over 2000 years and used as a specific for the nerves or the muscles.

Walnut (*Juglans nigra*—Black Walnut) hulls are used as a black or dark brown body or hair dye. The decoction of leaves is added to shampoos or bath herbs as an astringent, for skin disease such as herpes, and as an astringent mouthwash. In the *Doctrine of Signatures*, the Walnut perfectly represents the head, and all parts of it represent the various parts of the head. The oil is useful as a hot oil treatment for dry or dandruffy hair.

Watercress (*Nasturtium officinale*) is effective as a wash for blemishes and freckles.

Watermelon (*Citrullus vulgaris*) I spent a delightful year once hopping about a Watermelon field, following honeybees and observing their pollination habits on Watermelon blossoms. I can still recognize a female Watermelon flower at 10 paces and can still remember the delicious Watermelon juice facials I gave myself squatting out in the middle of the field hidden from view of the office. The meat of the Watermelon can be applied as a mask for normal skin and the juice is used as a facial water.

White Pond Lily (*Nymphaea odorata, Castalia odorata*) root and leaves decoction is an astringent demulcent wash for the legs or face and for inflamed or sore skin; it is used in lotions and creams.

Willow, White (*Salix alba*) bark is used in cosmetics because of its astringency and salicin content, which make it effective in the treatment of skin diseases such as eczema or herpes. It is also used in lotions, creams, and facial washes and as an ingredient in bath herb or facial herb mixtures. Mixed with Comfrey, mucilage of Quince, Ginseng, and tincture of Benzoin, it makes excellent emollient hydrating lotion for pimples or pussy bumps. The decoction of Patchouli, Thyme, and White Willow bark is an excellent deodorant wash. Infusion of White Willow and Lavender or Witch Hazel water makes an aftershave splash.

Wintergreen (*Gaultheria procumbens, Pyrola spp.*) contains methyl salicylate, which some people are very allergic to. It will *help* external skin problems as a decoction, but if you are sensitive to salicylates, it can also *cause* skin problems. The oil is obtained by water distillation; this means that the herb is intensely aromatic when used in bath herb or facial herb formulas. I love this smell and use the herb as often as possible. The plant can also be used as an astringent aromatic in lotions, creams, salves, and as a rub for arthritis, rheumatism, or sciatica. Its oil is used in flavors, candies, toothpaste, mouthwash, and cosmetics.

Wintersweet (*Chimonanthus fragrans,* also called *C. praecox*) Wintersweet is also another name for the herb Oregano. This has wonderfully scented yellow blossoms that can be infused in oil and used for massage or as a body oil. The flowers can be dropped into white wine to make a fragrant drink.

Witch Hazel (*Hamamelis virginiana*) bark and leaves are styptic, cleansing, and astringent, with a strong distinctive aromatic scent, have medicinal use, and are also added to soaps and cosmetics. An infusion or tea is an effective wash for the skin as an aftershave, rinse, or as a foot bath for aching tired feet, and for stings or sunburn. The decoction of the bark is used for inflamed skin or as a dandruff wash. The bark or leaf can be used as an aromatic astringent in lotions and creams, especially for oily skin; they can be added to bath herbs, hair rinses, or facial herb mixtures. A poultice of Witch Hazel and Comfrey is used for bruises, swollen surfaces, and varicose veins. As a skin tonic, it tightens loose tissue, is used for cellulite, and is an effective astringent tonic for red veins on the nose or face. Combined with Rosewater, Witch Hazel is a very soothing eyewash. In folklore a Witch Hazel branch is used to divine water. The extract is used for all the above purposes, for general all-around skin care, and as an underarm or genital deodorant.

WITCH HAZEL

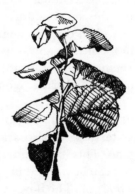

Woodruff (*Asperula odorata*) does not acquire its odor until dried, but it can be used either fresh or dried. It has a healing effect on superficial cuts and sores and is used in either facial herbs or bath herb mixtures. Also nice as an aftershave rinse or, when dried, in the last rinse cycle of your washing machine to scent your clothes.

☙ **Wormwood** (*Artemisia absinthium*) soaked in rum is used as a rub for fallen arches.

Yarrow (*Achillea millefolium*) is an astringent, mildly aromatic herb used for love-divining and stimulating hair growth. It is an active diaphoretic in bath herbs, a cleansing herb in facial mixtures, an astringent in vaginal douches (especially good if mixed with Comfrey and Mint), and is mixed in shampoo and hair potions for stimulating growth, eradicating dandruff, and eliminating unhealthy scalp conditions. It is also used as a mouthwash for toothache.

Yerba The Yerbas of California—Yerba Buena (*Satureja doglasii*), Yerba Mansa (*Anemopsis Californica*), and Yerba del Pasmo (*Adenostoma sparcifolium*)—are all used as cleansing washes for the skin, in bath herbs for aching muscles or tired feet, and as an external tea for skin infections.

Ylang-Ylang (*Cananga odorata, Canangium odoratum*) oil is produced in several places, one of which is the small island of Nossi-Bé off the coast of Madagascar. This oil is used in soapmaking and as a blender in perfumery. The ten-year-old tree produces about 20 pounds of flowers in a season, of which only two per cent is obtained in oil. The flowers can be infused in oil to make an interesting and delightful massage or body oil or hair oil. In fact, the flowers are rubbed directly on the hair as a hair dressing.

Yucca (*Yucca baccata, Y. spp.*) plant is quite beautiful, and its fragrant blossoms are used in California perfumery. Infused in oil, they are effective (smoothing) for body care; dropped into the bath they are a bath oil. The Yucca is one of the most famous soap plants of the American Southwest. The roots are scraped, mashed, mixed with water, rubbed into the hair or clothes, and then rinsed out. The soapy liquid can also be used as a cleansing wash for the skin.

Zdravetz (*Geranium macrorrhizum*) The name means "health" and the herb is used medicinally. The oil distilled in Bulgaria has some use in perfumery and soapmaking.

🌀 **Zinnia** (*Zinnea spp.*) is sometimes called the Mal de Ojo (sickness of the eye) because a hand that touches the flowers will carry irritants to the eye. It is used effectively as a hair rinse.

Some of the books referred to for Latin binomials: Arctander, Steffen. *Perfume and Flavour Materials of Natural Origin.* Elizabeth, New Jersey, 1960; Grieve, Mrs. M. *A Modern Herbal.* New York: Hafner Publishing Company, 1971 (originally published 1931); Hay, Roy and Patrick M. Synge. *The Color Dictionary of Flowers and Plants for Home and Garden.* New York: Crown Publishers in Collaboration with The Royal Horticultural Society, 1969; Neal, Marie C. *In Gardens of Hawaii.* Honolulu, Hawaii: Bernice P. Bishop Museum, Bishop Press, 1965; Nickell, J. M. *J. M. Nickell's Botanical Ready Reference.* Los Angeles, Calif.: M. L. Baker, 1972 (originally published 1911); Rickett, Harold William. *Wild Flowers of the United States.* New York: McGraw-Hill Book Co., 1971; Schery, Robert W. *Plants for Man,* 2nd edition. Englewood Cliffs, New Jersey: Prentice-Hall, Inc., 1972.

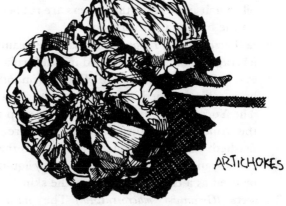

ARTICHOKES

"it mighta choked artie but it aint gonna choke me" - little rascals, 1930's

Chapter IV

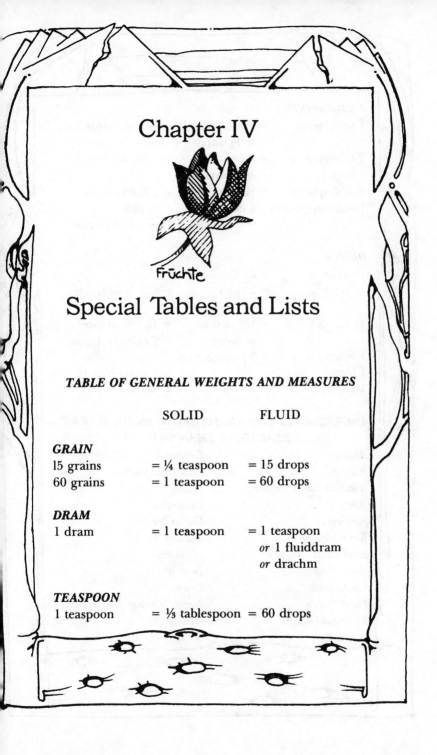

Früchte

Special Tables and Lists

TABLE OF GENERAL WEIGHTS AND MEASURES

	SOLID	FLUID
GRAIN		
15 grains	= ¼ teaspoon	= 15 drops
60 grains	= 1 teaspoon	= 60 drops
DRAM		
1 dram	= 1 teaspoon	= 1 teaspoon *or* 1 fluiddram *or* drachm
TEASPOON		
1 teaspoon	= ⅓ tablespoon	= 60 drops

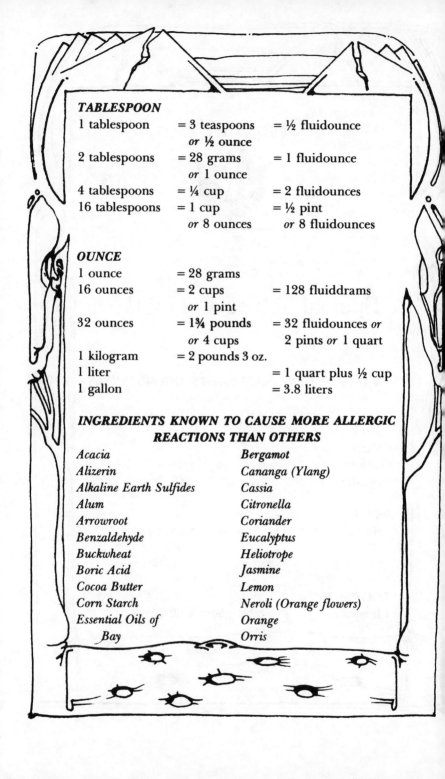

TABLESPOON

1 tablespoon	= 3 teaspoons	= ½ fluidounce
	or ½ ounce	
2 tablespoons	= 28 grams	= 1 fluidounce
	or 1 ounce	
4 tablespoons	= ¼ cup	= 2 fluidounces
16 tablespoons	= 1 cup	= ½ pint
	or 8 ounces	*or* 8 fluidounces

OUNCE

1 ounce	= 28 grams	
16 ounces	= 2 cups	= 128 fluiddrams
	or 1 pint	
32 ounces	= 1¾ pounds	= 32 fluidounces *or*
	or 4 cups	2 pints *or* 1 quart
1 kilogram	= 2 pounds 3 oz.	
1 liter		= 1 quart plus ½ cup
1 gallon		= 3.8 liters

INGREDIENTS KNOWN TO CAUSE MORE ALLERGIC REACTIONS THAN OTHERS

Acacia	*Bergamot*
Alizerin	*Cananga (Ylang)*
Alkaline Earth Sulfides	*Cassia*
Alum	*Citronella*
Arrowroot	*Coriander*
Benzaldehyde	*Eucalyptus*
Buckwheat	*Heliotrope*
Boric Acid	*Jasmine*
Cocoa Butter	*Lemon*
Corn Starch	*Neroli (Orange flowers)*
Essential Oils of	*Orange*
Bay	*Orris*

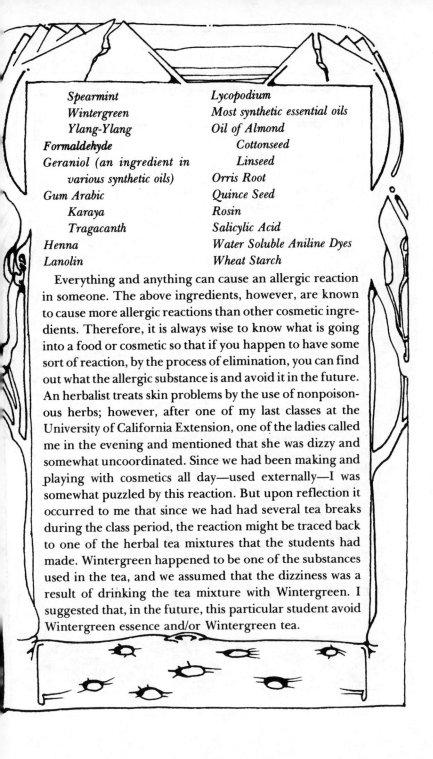

Spearmint
Wintergreen
Ylang-Ylang
Formaldehyde
Geraniol (an ingredient in
    various synthetic oils)
Gum Arabic
Karaya
Tragacanth
Henna
Lanolin

Lycopodium
Most synthetic essential oils
Oil of Almond
Cottonseed
Linseed
Orris Root
Quince Seed
Rosin
Salicylic Acid
Water Soluble Aniline Dyes
Wheat Starch

Everything and anything can cause an allergic reaction in someone. The above ingredients, however, are known to cause more allergic reactions than other cosmetic ingredients. Therefore, it is always wise to know what is going into a food or cosmetic so that if you happen to have some sort of reaction, by the process of elimination, you can find out what the allergic substance is and avoid it in the future. An herbalist treats skin problems by the use of nonpoisonous herbs; however, after one of my last classes at the University of California Extension, one of the ladies called me in the evening and mentioned that she was dizzy and somewhat uncoordinated. Since we had been making and playing with cosmetics all day—used externally—I was somewhat puzzled by this reaction. But upon reflection it occurred to me that since we had had several tea breaks during the class period, the reaction might be traced back to one of the herbal tea mixtures that the students had made. Wintergreen happened to be one of the substances used in the tea, and we assumed that the dizziness was a result of drinking the tea mixture with Wintergreen. I suggested that, in the future, this particular student avoid Wintergreen essence and/or Wintergreen tea.

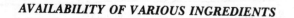

AVAILABILITY OF VARIOUS INGREDIENTS

Basic Ingredients—Available at Pharmacies (P) or Health Food Stores (HF)

P	Alcohol, rubbing and ethyl	HF	Henna
HF	Almond paste	HF	Herbs
P	Camphorated oil	HF	Honey
P	Castor oil	P	Lanolin
P	Cocoa butter	HF	Natural foods
P	Cod liver oil	HF	Natural grains
HF	Cold processed oils	HF	Natural vitamins
HF	Essential oils (usually synthetic)	P	Pumice stone
		HF	Sea salt
HF	Fruit kernel oils (almond, peach, apricot)	P	Talcum powder, unscented
		P	Tartaric acid
P	Fuller's earth	P	Tincture of benzoin
HF	Gelatin capsules	P	Witch Hazel
		P	Wood tar

Basic Ingredients—Available at Fine Department Stores or Health Food Stores

Brushes
  Natural boar bristle hair-brush
  Natural boar nailbrush
  Natural boar complexion brush

Gloves
  Cotton or kid
Loofahs
Natural sponges
Soaps

Basic Cosmetic Ingredients—Available at Herb Stores

Almond meal
Beeswax

Benzoin
Camphor

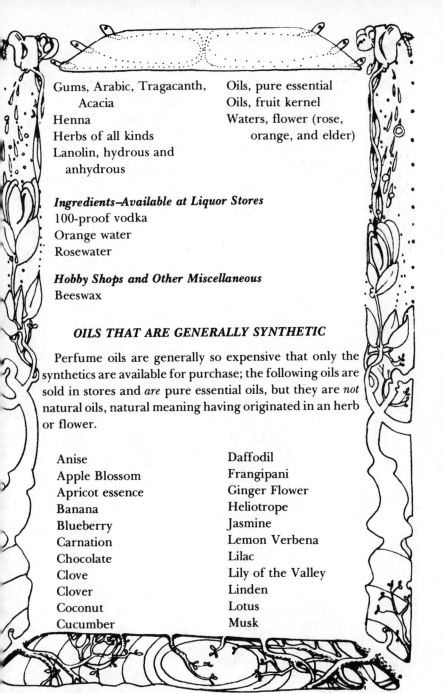

Gums, Arabic, Tragacanth, Acacia
Henna
Herbs of all kinds
Lanolin, hydrous and anhydrous

Oils, pure essential
Oils, fruit kernel
Waters, flower (rose, orange, and elder)

Ingredients—Available at Liquor Stores
100-proof vodka
Orange water
Rosewater

Hobby Shops and Other Miscellaneous
Beeswax

OILS THAT ARE GENERALLY SYNTHETIC

Perfume oils are generally so expensive that only the synthetics are available for purchase; the following oils are sold in stores and *are* pure essential oils, but they are *not* natural oils, natural meaning having originated in an herb or flower.

Anise
Apple Blossom
Apricot essence
Banana
Blueberry
Carnation
Chocolate
Clove
Clover
Coconut
Cucumber

Daffodil
Frangipani
Ginger Flower
Heliotrope
Jasmine
Lemon Verbena
Lilac
Lily of the Valley
Linden
Lotus
Musk

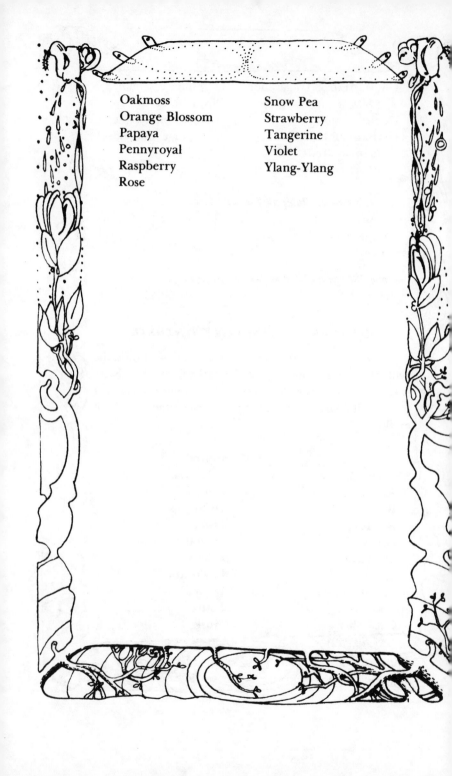

Oakmoss
Orange Blossom
Papaya
Pennyroyal
Raspberry
Rose

Snow Pea
Strawberry
Tangerine
Violet
Ylang-Ylang

Chapter V

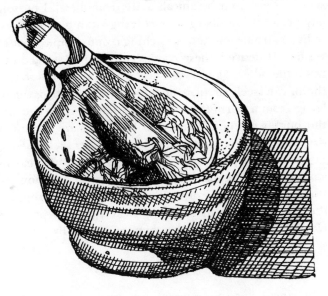

How to Collect, Use, and Store Cosmetic Plants and Equipment

COLLECTING OF PLANTS

ONLY COLLECT THOSE plants that you recognize; do not collect plants if you are unsure of their identity. Collect on a dry morning when the dew is dry on the plant and the sun is just high. Cut down your green herbs by a third; pluck your flowers; peel barks into thin strips. Then dry your plants; the green herbs can be tied in *small* bundles and hung in a cool, dry place, or *small* bunches can be wrapped in newspaper and placed near a slightly warm heater; they can also be placed loosely on a fiberglass

screen. Keep your botanicals away from metal. I personally prefer using fiberglass screening—can be purchased
in hardware stores—and stretching it onto simple wooden
frames. If desired, these frames can then be stacked one
upon the other. Flowers are best dried on screens so that
the air can freely circulate on both sides. Bark strips can be
hung from a warm dry ceiling and left there to age and
thoroughly dry out. When your botanicals are absolutely
dry, place them separately into brown paper sacks, *labeled*,
in a cool, dark place until ready for use. Or they may be
stored in airtight glass or metal containers. Additionally,
flowers can be made directly into tinctures by dropping
them immediately upon being picked into 50 per cent
alcohol or 100-proof vodka, rum, or Ng Ka Py.

STORING

Storing botanicals is easy—just keep them in clean,
labeled containers in cool, dark, and dry places. Plants are
delicate and lose their sterling qualities and beautiful color
if placed in the sun or on sunny shelves. Store them away,
check them occasionally for bugs, and if you find any,
discard the whole container of that herb by placing it in
your garden as mulch. If you find only a few bugs put the
entire container of herbs in your freezer for 3 days. The
cold kills the bugs and the larvae and the herbs can then be
used.

USING HERBS

Using herbs is great fun. Don't complicate matters by
thinking a particular mixture of herbs has only one use; in
fact, I make a mixture of herbs for steaming my skin and
use the same liquid not only as a beverage tea to drink, but
occasionally as a douche, both vaginal and nasal; then after
the face is steamed, the herbs are unceremoniously

dumped into a bathtub full of water and I take a bath. Afterwards I gather the herbs up from the water and place them in my garden where they proceed to mulch and nourish their living companions. See the glossary, Chapter II, for directions as to making infusions, tinctures, decoctions, etc. The beauty of making your own herbal cosmetics is that you use plants that have just been picked or freshly dried and so your cosmetics and preparations are absolutely fresh when you make them. Herbal infusions and decoctions will spoil with time, so when you make them, use the excess liquid to water your potted plants, as these solutions will nourish them as well as your skin.

The remainder of this book is composed of recipes made from DRIED herbs, except where indicated, but if you are fortunate enough to have fresh herbs by all means use them. One handful of dried herb is usually equal to two handfuls of fresh. One ounce of dried herb can be equal to 1 to 4 ounces of fresh depending on the quantity of water the fresh plant contains. For example, 1 ounce of dried Lettuce leaf is probably equal to 4 ounces or more of the fresh leaf, while 1 ounce of dried bark may be only 1¼ ounces of the fresh bark. Take all these things into consideration when you use herbs, but since the measurements are usually not at all critical, take pleasure in making the recipes and don't worry too much about the exactness of the measurements.

EQUIPMENT

Equipment consists of one or two different-sized enamel or nonmetal pots—one could be a double-boiler type or you can improvise a water bath; a few different sizes of wooden spoons; various sizes of glass bottles and jars for holding the finished product; a simple table-top scale to weigh the various ingredients; measuring spoons; a couple of small enamel bowls; a mortar and pestle; and if you wish, a blender and a seed grinder. Here is a list of equipment:

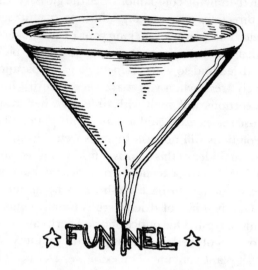

☆ FUNNEL ☆

Bowls of various sizes
Cheesecloth for straining
Containers for creams and
   liquids
Enamel double boiler
Enamel pots and pans
Funnels
Jars
Measuring cups and
   spoons

Mortar and pestle
Muslin for straining
Postal scale
Weighing scale
Wooden spoons

Optional equipment
   Blender
   Seed or coffee bean
      grinder

Chapter VI

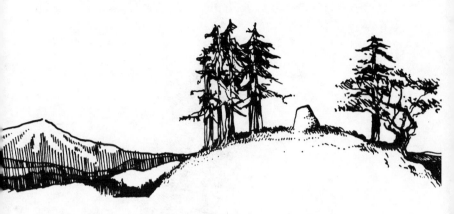

Where in the World to Buy Your Basic Ingredients, Your Herbs, or If You're Lazy, the Finished Product

NOWADAYS THERE MUST be many, many stores in the United States, Canada, and the rest of the world that sell herbs and excellent organic natural cosmetics. Check in the Yellow Pages of your telephone directory and with your friends for their favorite stores. Try the listings under:

Botanicals
Health Food Stores
Herbs
Nature or Natural Ingre-
    dients
Oils, Animal
Oils, Essential

Perfumes
Pharmacies, Natural or
    Homeopathic
Raw Materials
Sachets
Soaps
Spices

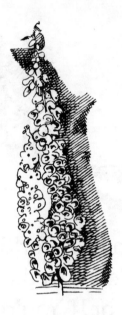

For fine, reasonably priced cosmetics, kid gloves, and boar bristle hairbrushes, check health food and fine department stores.

CALIFORNIA

When you shop, watch the cosmetics, though, as there are now a lot of unscrupulous companies putting out so-called natural cosmetics that really aren't. Make sure the cosmetics *list all* ingredients. So read those labels and determine for yourself what is best.

Earth Beam Natural Foods, Burlingame

Earth Sign Natural Foods, Menlo Park

Esalen Institute, Big Sur

> Has a delightful selection of massage oils available that you can use along with your mental and psychic therapy.

Felton International Inc., 2242 Purdue Avenue, Los Angeles, California 90064
  Sells flavors, fragrances, essential oils, and aromatics, generally in large quantities only.

Hathaway Allied Products, 24002 Frampton Avenue, Harbor City, California 90710
  Sells herbs and gums, generally in larger quantities than is needed or wanted by most individuals.

Herb Products Company, 11012 Magnolia Boulevard, North Hollywood, California 91601
  Also known as Living Herbs. One of the better large herb stores. Has herbs, spices, tinctures, essential oils, and many Ginseng products. Write for a catalog.

Naked Scent, 813 State Street, Santa Barbara, California 93101
  Carries many fine herbal products including a complete selection of massage and body oils.

Nature's Herb Company, 281 Ellis Street, San Francisco, California 94102
  Still the most economical, but now unfortunately, the busiest place around. Please don't ask to buy by the spoonsful. Order by the ounce, quarter-pound, or more. But this goes for all herb stores. They sell herbs, potpourri ingredients, and other basic cosmetic supplies. A catalog is available. This is still my favorite store; the people are knowledgeable, and the herbs the best.

New Age Creations—Herbal Cosmetics, 219 Carl Street, San Francisco, California 94117
  Massage and body oils, herbal shampoos and rinses, bath herbs, sleep pillows, facials, herbal body powders, potpourris, etc. All products made with herbs, and the ingredients are listed on the label. Catalog 25 ¢.

San Francisco Herb and Natural Food Co., P.O. Box 40604, San Francisco, California 94103, and 113 Alder Street, West Babylon, New York 11704

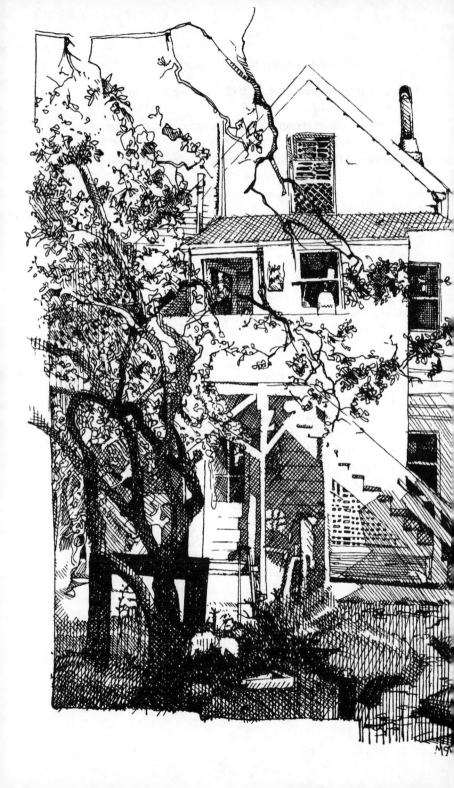

Carries a full line of herbs. The quality is uneven but generally good to superior. They sell both retail and wholesale. An Herb Guide that comes with your catalog is very useful.

Star Herb Company, 38 Miller Avenue, Mill Valley, California 94941

Carries a complete line of herbs and herbal products including *cosmetics* and tea blends. They also carry occasionally, PURE essential oils that are very difficult to get elsewhere. A catalog is available and they sell both retail and wholesale.

Sunflower Natural Foods, 821 41st Avenue, Santa Cruz, California 90670

Superior Trading Company, 867 Washington Street, San Francisco, California 94108

Ginseng, Ginseng, and more Ginseng. Super quality and very fair prices.

Thom's Natural Food, 843 Clement Street, San Francisco, California 94118

A very good selection of food, food ingredients for delicious cosmetics, a fine array of books, and a selection of herbal cosmetics.

Tillotson's Roses, Brown's Valley Road, Watsonville, California 95076

This is the nursery in California and on the West Coast to order your old Roses for the making of real old-fashioned potpourris, and the Roses you will need for the creation of your own Rosewater, Rose oil, and other cosmetic Rose creations. A beautiful catalog is available.

Tlaloc Botanic Foods, P.O. Box 46312, Los Angeles, California 90046, and **Yerbas Sierra Madre,** Colonia Juarez, Chihuahua, Mexico

A limited but excellent selection of high-quality Mexican herbs. Write for a catalog and try the delicious Pericón Tea.

CONNECTICUT

Hemlock Hill Herb Farm, Litchfield, Connecticut 06759

Grows medicinal and aromatic herbs and sells a few plants generally unavailable elsewhere, such as Orris and the Egyptian Top Onion.

Truc International, Inc., Box 167, Woodstock Hill, Connecticut 06281

An absolutely fantastic array of absolutely fantastic soaps from all over the world. These are distributed all over the country and the companies represented include Crabtree & Evelyn of London, meal soaps, Puhls of Berlin, fruit and flower soaps, F. Wolff & Sohn, incomparable flower soaps, Monpelas of Paris, English Coal Tar soap (Wright's), and other cosmetic products including creams, lotions, and bath accessories. If you have tender or sensitive skin try Neca 7 or Swiss Buttermilk or Sinalca. They may be wholesale only but look for their soaps in fine stores everywhere.

ILLINOIS

Herbarium, Inc., 2019 West Iowa Street, Chicago, Illinois 60622, or Route 2, Box 620, Kenosha, Wisconsin 53140

Imports and exports botanical drugs and spices generally in quantities too large to be of use to the average-at-home cosmetic maker.

INDIANA

Indiana Botanic Gardens, Inc., Hammond, Indiana 46325

An excellent herb store, it has a mail-order department, sells all basic cosmetic ingredients including herbal cosmetics and castile soap powder for shampoos.

KANSAS

Cook's Geranium Nursery, 712 North Grand, Lyons, Kansas 67554
Sells Geraniums for you to grow into large plants for Geranium cosmetics.

MARYLAND

Carroll Gardens, Westminster, Maryland 21157
Sells native live plants.

MASSACHUSETTS

Organic Food Cellar, 297a Newbury Street, Boston, Massachusetts 02115, or 31 Putnam Avenue, Cambridge, Massachusetts 02139
Good selection of foods, natural ingredients useful in cosmetics, and some really nice herbal cosmetics.

MICHIGAN

Harvest Health, Inc., 1944 Eastern Avenue, S.E., Grand Rapids, Michigan 49507
Harry E. Saier, Dimondale, Michigan 48821
Dishcloth Gourd seeds, among others. Also the Sponge Gourd, *Luffa Cylindrica*.

MISSISSIPPI

Carl Odom, Pinola, Mississippi 39149
Sells Dishcloth Gourd seeds, and lots of other Gourds and seeds.

MISSOURI

Luyties Pharmacal Company, 4200 Laclede Avenue, St. Louis, Missouri 63108
A homoeopathic pharmacy.

NEW JERSEY

Meer Corporation, North Bergen, New Jersey 07047
Sells herbs, tinctures, spices, essential oils, and related botanical products, but only in large quantities.

NEW YORK

Anthroposophic Press, Inc., 258 Hungry Hollow Road, Spring Valley, New York 10977
Send for their small catalog of books dealing mainly with Anthroposophy, that school of thought devised by Rudolf Steiner, and whose definition absolutely defies me. I am particularly fond of their books dealing with child care, such as *Brothers and Sisters* by Karl Koenig and *Conception, Birth and Early Childhood* by Norbert Glas.

Aphrodisia, 28 Carmine Street, New York, New York 10014
My goodness, what an incredible lot of herbal goodies; herbs, herb books, tea blends, culinary herb mixtures, herbal mixtures from other lands but alas, no herbal cosmetics. One dollar will buy their mail-order catalog, which is more than a catalog, a delightful book of herbs.

Boyd Chemists, Inc., 655 Madison Avenue, New York, New York 10021
On my last trip to New York I stopped in this store and was amazed at the varied amount of make-up and the girls deftly making up everyone in sight with tons

and gobs of goo. Having successfully bypassed the witty and one tart-tongued make-up girl I found the bins of natural boar bristle brushes and walls of intriguing cosmetic equipment. It was great fun shopping there and definitely a worthwhile visit.

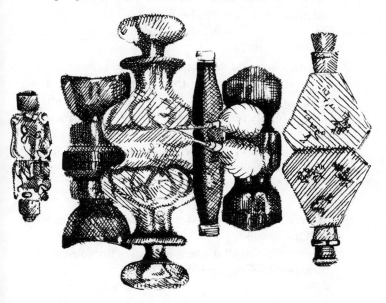

Caswell-Massey Company, Lexington Avenue and 48th Street, New York, New York 10017, Catalog Order Department, 320 West 13th Street, New York, New York 10014

A fantastic pharmacy, carries basic ingredients for homemade cosmetics, a large selection of cosmetics, basic potpourri ingredients, as well as a wonderful array of soaps. A good selection of natural bristle brushes and other herbal delights.

Kiehl Pharmacy, 109 Third Avenue, New York, New York 10003

Still one of my favorite pharmacies. It's too bad they don't mail order. But if you are in New York don't fail to stop in. They sell herbs for cosmetics, *pure* essential oils, and their own perfumes.

United Communications, Box 320, Woodmere, New York 11598

Send for their catalog of botanical prints and their complicated, incredible herb guide.

Weleda, Inc., 30 South Main Street, Spring Valley, New York 10977

A high-minded company that only sells cosmetic preparations made from the finest ingredients. The products are marvelous—I have tried most of them and can highly recommend *all* the baby care products and all the Calendula cosmetics. They have "books by Rudolf Steiner, concerned with the hygienic-therapeutic aspects of Anthroposophy."

OHIO

Joseph Kern Rose Nursery, Department H, Box 33, Mentor, Ohio 44060

Grow and sell all the best old Roses for your use in cosmetics. Catalog available.

OREGON

Atlantis Rising, 7915 S. E. Stark, Portland, Oregon 97215

An incredible catalog loaded with all manner of goodies: herbs and spices; articles on Ginseng, Fo-ti-tieng, Gotu Kola, Dong Kwai, and Golden Seal (rejuvenative herbs all); herbal formulas for many ailments; a large and grand variety of herbal cosmetics; herb seeds; occult oils; herbal capsules and tea blends and a grand variety of books.

Nichols Garden Nursery, 1190 North Pacific Highway, Albany, Oregon 97321

Ah, the joys of elephant Garlic. It took me two years to get my order from Nichols because the demand is so great—but finally I received ten 1-ounce cloves, planted them, and this summer harvested my crop of 1-pound bulbs. Very mild tasting. Garlic should be eaten every day for health as well as a beautiful complexion. The catalog is free and full of herb plants, seeds, and all sorts of basic ingredients.

PENNSYLVANIA

Haussman's Pharmacy, 6th and Girard Avenue, Philadelphia, Pennsylvania 19127
All sorts of herbal mixtures, ingredients, and herbs.
Penn Herb Company, 603 North 2nd Street, Philadelphia, Pennsylvania 19123
So far this is the only place I have found that lists nonanimal gelatin capsules in their catalog. Sells lots of herbs and books. Get their catalog; it is definitely a must.

RHODE ISLAND

Greene Herb Garden, Greene, Rhode Island 02898
Herb seeds and bulbs.
Meadowbrook Herb Garden, Wyoming, Rhode Island 02898
Herbal everything including herbs, teas, cosmetics, Wala Elixirs that are an indispensable nutritional aid, and of course those wonderful herbal cosmetics by Dr. R. Hauschka.

TEXAS

Ault Bee Farms, Weslaco, Texas 78596
Sells honey, royal jelly, and *Aloe vera* by the pound.
Good Food Store, 1101 West 5th Street, Austin, Texas 78703

Natural foods, grains, all those natural food ingredients for delicious cosmetics.

Hilltop Herb Farm, Box 866, Cleveland, Texas 77327

Herbs, herb plants, delicious meals, books, and scented Geraniums. Catalog 30¢.

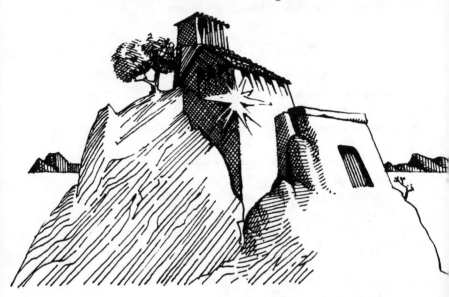

UTAH

Whole Earth Natural Foods, 1026 2nd Avenue, Salt Lake City, Utah 84103

Natural foods and natural food ingredients for beautiful cosmetics, as well as a supply of natural herbal cosmetics.

WISCONSIN

Herbarium, Inc., Kenosha, Wisconsin 53140

North Central Comfrey Producers, Box 195B, Glidden, Wisconsin 54527

Sells Comfrey plants.

The Soap Opera, 312 State Street, Madison, Wisconsin 53703

Has an excellent assortment of cosmetics and herbal cosmetics. They sell books, and this might be the place to try for those excellent Truc soaps.

Woodland Acres Nursery, Route 2, Highway W, Crivetz, Wisconsin 54114

Specialize in Ferns and wild flowers, many of which have herbal cosmetic use.

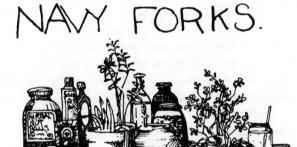

CANADA

Wide World of Herbs Ltd., 11 Saint Catherine Street East, Montreal 129, Quebec, Canada

Lots and lots of different herbs including some that I have seen nowhere else. Also an extensive dye herb catalog. Many essential oils, including *real* oil of Cardamon, and Neroli Natural ($184.80/oz.), and the only catalog that I have ever seen that sells and lists Rose Otto True Type ($212.80/oz.).

ENGLAND

Culpepper Limited, 21 Bruton Street, London, England

Wonderful herbal lotions, soaps, toilet water, bath

preparations, hair preparations, eyelash grower, herbs and spices for cooking, herbs, medicinal herbal blends, pills and tablets, exquisite herbal creams, ointments, lotions, and all manner of everything herbal. The catalog can be had for 25 cents. Above the shop is the London Herbal Treatment Centre where there are consultant herbalists for medical problems.

New Age Creations—Herbal Cosmetics by Vivian, 31 Clarendon Gardens, London W9, England.

OTHERS

Weleda Herbal Cosmetics was founded in Switzerland in 1912 to answer a demand for natural medicines and treatment preparations. These products continue to be made by people rather than machines, mainly from herbs grown bio-dynamically. They are available in every major country in the Western world.

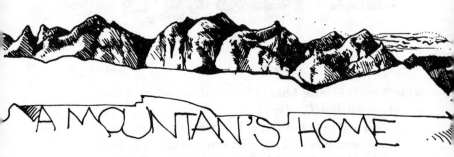

HERBAL SCHOOLS AND GROUPS

I can't really say much about the curriculum of the schools since I have not attended any of them. Some will not send their texts unless a fee is paid and so it is impossible to do anything but give an address and hope that you will use your best judgment in deciding whether or not their programs are worth the enrollment. They are listed without order.

Herb Walks with Nan Koehler, 1682 Indian Valley Road, Novato, California 94947. $2.00 donation.

Emerson Institute of Herbology, 815 Bancroft Street, Pointe Claire, Quebec, Canada. $175.00 for a home-study course in Herbology.

See Institute, 14016 Armstrong Woods Road, Guerneville, California 95446. Various programs and herbal retreats at a very reasonable sum.

University of California Extension, 55 Laguna Street, San Francisco, California 94102 and Campus, Santa Cruz, California 95064. Send for a catalog of their wonderful classes—including herbal studies classes taught by this author. $40 to $75.

The Institute of Herbal Philosophy, 115 E. Foothill, Glendora, California 91740. Mail-order course for $52.50.

Dominion Herbal College, 7527 Kingsway, Burnaby 3, British Columbia, Canada. Mail-order course for about $150.00.

School of Natural Healing, P.O. Box 352, Provo, Utah 84601. Mail-order course for about $75.00.

Part II
THE RECIPES

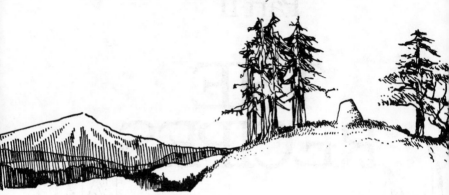

. . . UNCOMMON PAINS have been taken to improve
the present Edition, which contains a System of the Cosmetic Art, infinitely superior to any that has hitherto ap-
peared; and it has likewise uniformly rendered the various
Prescriptions not only compatible with, but subservient to
the Preservation, and even the Improvement of Health; an
Object of the greatest Importance in a Work of this Kind.

This was first written in a knowledgeable work called *The
Toilet of Flora*, published in 1779. *The Toilet* is a book devoted to the use of herbs and natural substances as cosmetics, for men as well as women, to improve the body
rather than to just cover up its imperfections; in fact, it is
an Herbal Body Book—as this book is entitled and meant
to be.

F IS FOR FACE

An attractive complexion is primarily a result of perfect nutrition, proper cleansing, and exercise. Your skin mirrors the health of your body, indicating, by dark circles under the eyes or sallow color, improper treatment. If you feel good and rest well, it is bound to show up in healthy-looking skin. However, in this polluted nervous world, it is sometimes difficult to keep our skin clean and healthy looking by using just ordinary soap and water every day.

The late Adelle Davis, my favorite nutritionist, has written several books on what to eat. Look at *Let's Eat Right to Keep Fit* for hints on healthy eating. *Prevention Magazine* is also a good source of nutritional information.

Perfect cleansing with herbal and other natural substances is easily accomplished and results in skin that looks clean and doesn't need sticky, camouflaging cosmetics to look good. You can wash your face with soap and water every morning and every night. Use whatever soap suits you best—it isn't necessary to use neutral or acid types. Indeed, dermatologists have found that acid soaps are no better or worse for the skin than alkaline soaps. My skin responds better to high quality alkaline soaps, such as pure castile, than to acid soaps such as Amino-Pon. These acid soaps dry me out and make my skin feel tight and itchy. Occasionally I use neutral soaps such as Neca 7 or Sinalca for a pleasant change.

HOW TO WASH YOUR FACE

First *wet* your face with warm water; you want to fill up the pores and relax them a little. Then with a bar of soap work up some lather in your *hands* and apply the lather to your face. A *little* facial massage is good at this point. Lather your face in circular upward and outward movements, up and around the throat, the chin, the nose, and the eyes. The lather picks up the dirt in the pores and then a rinse with lots of warm water washes it away. End up with a splash of cool water or a spray of mineral water, such as Evian, to cool and contract the pores.

Daily cleansing is important. If your skin is extra dry you may want to forego an occasional skin shampoo in favor of deep pore cleansing by herbal steam. In any case learn to recognize what type of skin you have. There are no overnight miracles for a beautiful complexion; skin must be

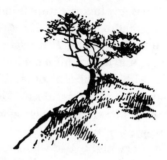

cared for every day. I prefer a daily washing with soap, twice a week steaming with my Extra Special Herbal Facial formula, and a once a week herbal mask.

THREE STEPS TO HANDSOME, CLEAR SKIN

1. A relaxing aroma massage especially for pimples and troubled skin to soothe the skin, ease tension, and calm the nerves.
2. An herbal steam to open the pores.
3. An herbal mask to nourish, tighten, and then maybe a Honey Pat good enough to eat for the dry patches.

DRY SKIN is usually thin and so delicate that there seems to be no openings for the pores; it looks old with many little lines, especially around the eyes. Soap and water washing, although necessary, should be followed with a soothing emollient or else the dry skin feels tight. Extremely rich or greasy creams are not good for dry skin. In fact, the application of these creams makes the skin lazy; it often completely stops producing its own oil. Hydrate dry skin with natural ingredients that supply extra moisture such as honey and herbs. Use simple moisturizers such as mucilage of flax.

OLD SKIN is also often thin and delicate and needs extra moisturizing. It looks saggy and lacks moisture but should not be overmassaged. Application of vitamin E formulas with honey works wonders on old skin. The pores occasionally become enlarged and coarse and here buttermilk facials are most useful. Again, rich greasy creams strangle and suffocate the pores. Use a gentle hand with facials and cosmetics and keep to the natural nourishing types of food both for your insides and outsides.

OILY SKIN looks shiny, thick, and coarse, often with enlarged pores. Do not use alcohol astringents, as they only further coarsen the texture of the skin. Diluted lemon juice and herbal waters are helpful for refining texture. Improperly washed, oily skin seems to get more oily and breaks out in blemishes and blackheads. Rejoice if you have oily skin as it ages well, developing less wrinkles and lines than dry skin.

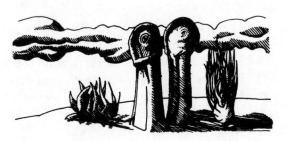

Chapter VII

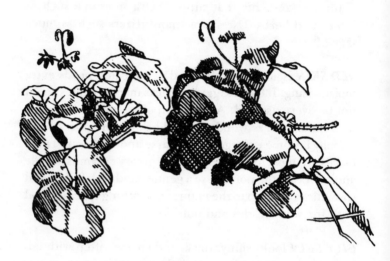

Facial Steaming
for Perfect Cleansing

THE ORIENTAL ARTICHOKE

EVERYONE CAN have a clear skin—skin that is pore-deep clean—without any special equipment or a great deal of money. All it takes is a towel, some herbs, a nonmetal pot with a top and some water, pure spring or distilled water if you have it but city water will do too. (If you have the time, take a gallon of your city water and let it sit in an open bottle for 24 hours to get rid of the chlorine.)

BASIC STEAMING DIRECTIONS

1. Carefully and gently wash your face and leave it moist.
2. Drop 2 tablespoons of herbs into the pot, add about 1 quart of water, cover the pot with the top.
3. Set the pot on a medium fire and bring to a boil, lower the heat, and *simmer* the herbs for about 3 minutes to extract all their wonderful, cleansing, medicating, volatile essences.
4. Now, turn off the heat, and remove the pot to a table.
5. Cover your hair with a cap or turban or tie it back.
6. With a bath towel cover your head and the pot (make a towel tent), and then remove the lid of the pot. Let the steam come up straight into your face. If your skin is delicate or if the veins are close to the surface, back away from the pot so that your skin doesn't get too hot and overstimulated. In any case you should be about 8 inches away from the pot. Let this herbal steam play about your face with your eyes closed for about 10 minutes, turning your face back and forth. When the steam starts to cool, I blow into it to get a better blast onto any problem areas.
7. You must remember that steaming greatly opens the pores, ridding the skin of toxins and impurities, and so you must follow your steaming by rinsing with warm and then cool water, or by splashing with an astringent to "close" the pores. Since it takes time for the pores to fully contract I would suggest that you stay inside for about an hour or so.

Herbal steaming cleans naturally, increases perspiration thereby deep cleaning every pore completely, and removes dirt, leftover cosmetics, and that nasty residue that dirty air and soot leave on the skin. Steaming hydrates by adding moisture, increases circulation, and has the added benefit of relieving tension. Your skin will look younger, more vibrant and alive because the circulation will have been improved. When I am particularly tired and feel all yellow and sallow, 5 minutes of an herbal steam cleaning followed by a Honey Pat, and I am a new woman (the Oriental Artichoke once again).

If your face is very dirty with many clogged pores you can give yourself 2 or 3 facial steams in succession. Then after that, 2 to 3 times a week or even less should be sufficient. Too much steam or steaming too often can remove the natural skin moisture and the essential skin oils. So use it in moderation and never act as if steaming or any other herbal treatment is totally harmless.

There are many types of recipes one can formulate for steaming different types of skin. Basically you will want to use a mixture of ⅓ "Licorice" herbs for removing impurities, ⅓ healing herbs like Comfrey, and ⅓ stimulating or soothing herbs like Mint or Camomile.

NORMAL TO DRY SKIN

Mix together equal quantities of Licorice root-PO[1], Fennel-PO, Camomile-WH, Clover-CS, Comfrey root-PO, and Comfrey leaf-CS. Use about 2 tablespoons of this mixture per steaming, following the basic directions, and store the excess herbs in a covered light-proof container.

OILY TO NORMAL SKIN

Lemon peel-CS, Lemongrass-CS, Roses-WH, Witch Hazel leaves or Bark-CS, and Lavender-WH, are all useful herbs for oily skin, so a mixture of any one or several of these

[1]PO—powdered, CS—cut and sifted, WH—whole.

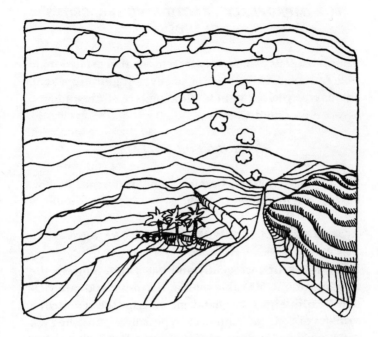

herbs with an equal quantity of Fennel and Comfrey would make an excellent steaming mixture.

ACNE STEAM

A mixture of Lavender, Licorice, and Comfrey root.

TIGHTENING STEAM, VERY STIMULATING

Peppermint-CS, Anise seed-PO, Lavender-WH, and Comfrey leaf-CS. Follow the basic directions.

STIMULATING STEAM

Mix equal quantities of Nettle, Rosemary, Fennel, and Peach leaves or Pansy leaves.

FOR IMPROPERLY FUNCTIONING SEBACEOUS GLANDS

Your sebaceous glands (they secrete oil), if not functioning well, can create either a dry or an oily condition of the skin. In this case you will want to use a mixture of Lemongrass, Licorice root, and Comfrey.

FORMULA FOR ECZEMA

Pansy, Violet flowers, Comfrey root, and White Willow bark; equal quantities of each.

FORMULA FOR WRINKLES OR DRY SKIN

First wash your face gently and pat it dry. Squeeze the contents of one 500-unit vitamin E capsule and one vitamin A capsule into your hand and massage the oils into the wrinkles of your face and neck, especially around the eyes and nose. Then steam with a mixture of Dandelion, Comfrey, Cowslip, Camomile, and Licorice. Orange blossoms are a terrific addition if you can get fresh blossoms.

JEANNE ROSE'S EXTRA SPECIAL SOOPER DOOPER HERBAL FACIAL FORMULA
For Any Kind of Skin or Combination of Problems

1 oz. of each of the following herbs in cut form:

Dandelion leaf	Peppermint
Camomile	Lavender
Pansy	Roses
Violet flowers	Dulse
Anise seed	Lettuce
Licorice root	Lemongrass
Fennel seed	Peach leaf
Caraway seed	Red clover

As you can see this makes 1 lb. of herbs, enough to last a very long time. I also use this mixture as a steam for a sore throat or tonsils and it isn't a bad beverage tea either.

THE ORIENTAL ARTICHOKE

It's been said that Alice, my husband's wife, has prickly pointy outsides but soft and mushy insides. Here is her favorite mixture of herbs for a quick steam: Artichoke leaves, Comfrey leaves, Fennel seed, and Peppermint leaves.

THE SAN CLEMENTE ORANGE STEAM

Very soothing and hydrating. Mix together equal quantities of Orange peel, Orange flowers, Fennel, Comfrey root, and Marshmallow root.

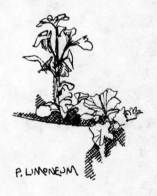

P. LIMONEUM

Chapter VIII

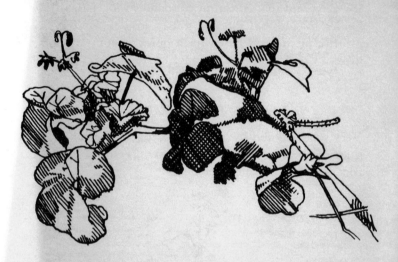

Lotions, Potions and Pores, Creams and Moisturizers

THERE IS NO substitute for a good diet to balance the functions of your skin but if your diet is good and you still feel the need for a cream, there are dozens of lotions, night creams, day creams, moisturizers, or just plain creams that one can formulate using herbs to aid this balance. Basically you have to figure out just what you want the cream to do, find the herbs to do the job (Chapter VI), and then make your cream. A properly formulated cream or lotion can be used on face, body, hands—male or female, adult or child. If the ingredients are edible and fit to eat, then they are probably good enough for your skin.

A lotion and a cream are basically the same thing, but the cream contains more solidifiers such as lanolin or beeswax. Lotions and creams can be made astringent, emollient, drying, tonic, stimulating, antiseptic, moisturizing, lubricating, aromatic, or hydrating according to the plant from which it is made.

A basic cream would have a formula as follows:

BASIC CREAM

1½ oz. solidifier and/or solid fat such as: 1 oz. lanolin *and* ½ oz. beeswax

3–4 oz. skin oil such as: 2 oz. Almond oil *and* 2 oz. Soy oil

1 oz. herb water such as: 1 oz. Rosewater

5 drops essential oil (1 drop/oz. optional) such as: 5 drops oil of Rose

Melt the solidifier and/or solid fat together in the top of an enamel double boiler or in a small enamel pot. Add the oils a bit at a time, stirring continuously. Turn off the heat and slowly add the herbed water, again stirring continuously until the cream has cooled. Add the essential oil and stir it in completely. Spoon or pour into a 6-oz. jar, labeled as to the contents. The jar should be opaque such as the old-fashioned milk glass or amber glass. You can also use clear glass by covering the jar with some type of colored paper.

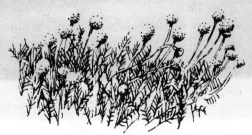

BASIC LOTION

1 oz. solidifier or solid fat such as: 1 oz. lanolin *or* Cocoa butter	2 oz. herb water: 2 oz. Rosewater
3 oz. skin oil: 3 oz. Almond *or* vegetable oil	5 drops essential oil (optional): 5 drops oil of Rose

Melt the solidifier and/or solid fat together in the top of an enamel double boiler or in a small enamel pot. Add the oil and the herb water alternately, a bit at a time, stirring continuously. Remove the pot from the heat. Add the essential oil and stir it in completely. Pour into a small, 6–8-oz. opaque glass or plastic bottle. Shake the bottle almost continuously until the lotion has cooled.

As you can see from the above recipes the equipment necessary for making your creams is minimal. A small enamel pot, a wooden spoon, measuring cup, measuring spoons, and a container for the finished product are all that are needed.

Now that we know how to make a basic cream it is easy to go from here to the made-to-personal-skin-type-order sort of cream.

AGING SKIN CREAM

1½ oz. lanolin—or Cocoa butter if you are allergic to lanolin.

(I always use anhydrous lanolin when making my cosmetics but hydrous lanolin, already having water added to it, can also be used. Simply reduce the amount of other liquid in the recipe.)

4 oz. Avocado oil

1 oz. Comfrey root water (Simmer 1 oz. cut Comfrey root in 2 cups of water in a covered nonmetal pot for 20 minutes. Or simmer it in the top of a double boiler for 20 minutes, let it cool, and then strain through muslin or cheesecloth.)

Follow the Basic Cream directions.

MOISTURIZING VITAMIN E CREAM

4 oz. Olive oil	5000 units vitamin E
3 T. beeswax	5 drops oil of Orange
2 oz. Orange water	flower or Orange peel

Melt the oil and the wax in the top of an enamel or glass double boiler, remove from heat, add your Orange water, and stir thoroughly. Pierce 10 capsules of 500 units of vitamin E and squeeze the contents into the cream. Add your essential oil and stir continuously until cool. This cream is very moisturizing and emollient. It is quite nice for rough, dry, or chapped complexions and should help to promote healthy-looking skin.

COLD CREAM FOR CLEANSING

The simplest cleansing cream in the world is made by adding 1 oz. of Olive oil to 4 oz. of Crisco and adding 5–10 drops of compound tincture of Benzoin. Apply your cream to a damp, washed face in upward spiraling movements. Massage in circles with the balls of your fingers around the nose, cheeks, and forehead, always moving in upward, outward movements. Then, lie on a slant board or at least raise your legs with a few pillows and stay relaxed for a few minutes—20 if you have the time. Remove the cream with tissues and either completely remove the residue with an astringent or leave the residue on overnight as skin food to be removed in the morning.

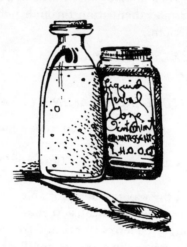

NOURISHING SKIN FOOD

Simmer 1 oz. of each of the following herbs: Camomile for puffiness, Orange peel as an antiseptic, Comfrey root as a cell regenerative, and Pansy for skin disease, in 2 cups of water in a covered nonmetal pot for 20 minutes. Strain out the herbs and use them as a facial mask or dump them into the garden to nourish your plants as compost. Melt 4 oz. of anhydrous lanolin and ½ oz. beeswax and add the herb water, beating constantly; now add Orange oil, about 1 t. Beat until cold and set. Keep this in the fridge where it should last about 1 week and maybe much longer. Use it every night and every morning.

MILK AND HONEY LOTION

Melt some honey and add an equal amount of skim milk. Honey is an humectant in that it draws moisture out of the air so it is within reach of the pores. Apply the milk and honey to your face or bosom, massage gently, take a warm bath or shower and rinse it off.

AVOCADO MINT ACTIVATOR

Macerate some fresh Mint in a blender or with a mortar and pestle. Add an equal quantity of ripe Avocado and blend together thoroughly. Wash your face and leave it slightly damp. Apply the Avocado Mint Activator, massaging it into the skin with the usual upward and outward movements, but in this case use the Avocado pit to do the massaging. Massage for a few minutes. Remove the excess cream with tissue and rinse with mint water or tea as an astringent.

OILY SKIN LOTION

Use either Witch Hazel extract or Lavender water, 1 cup, and soak 1 T. Quince seed in the liquid until it forms a gel. Apply this as a cleansing cream or an aftershave lotion.

ROSEWATER CREAM For Dry Skin

½ oz. beeswax	½ oz. Rosewater
2 oz. Olive oil	½ oz. Sweet Almond oil

Use the same directions as for the Basic Cream.

A COSMETIC JUICE

"*The Toilet of Flora*; or, A Collection of the Most Simple and Approved Methods of Preparing Baths, Essences, Pomatums, Powders, Perfumes, and Sweet-Scented Waters. With Receipts for Cosmetics of every Kind, that can smooth and brighten the Skin, give Force to Beauty, and take off the Appearance of Old Age and Decay. For the Use of the Ladies" was originally printed in MDCCLXXIX or 1779 in London. It is a marvelous book with many delightful recipes for beauty. Before going to bed or before or after you apply a cleansing cream, apply the following complexion brightener:

Make a hole in a Lemon, fill it with Sugar Candy (rock sugar, the kind that comes on a string), and close it nicely with leaf Gold (you could also use aluminum foil) applied over the rind that was cut out; then roast the Lemon in hot ashes. When desirous of using the juice, squeeze out a little through the hole, and wash the face with a napkin wetted with it. This juice effectively cleanses the skin, and brightens the complexion.

BEAN FLOWER CREAM *For Any Type Skin*

To a pint of cream add a handful of Bean flowers and simmer this ever so gently in the top of a double boiler for 15 minutes. Let it cool and strain through absolutely clean cheesecloth. Keep this lotion in the fridge and use it to refresh your skin, especially on hot summer days.

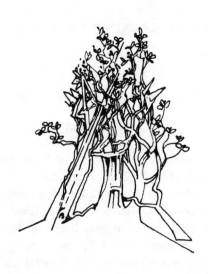

CHAPPED SKIN LOTION

1 T. borax	3 oz. glycerin
12 oz. double Rosewater	5 T. mucilage of Quince

Shake together the borax and the Rosewater until the borax is dissolved; add the mucilage of Quince to the glycerin and shake together until thoroughly incorporated; mix the 2 solutions together until well integrated.

HONEYDEW CREAM For Dry Skin

Mash with a mortar and pestle some Honeydew Melon. Strain the mashed mess through some cheesecloth to get 1 oz. of juice. Melt ½ oz. beeswax or lanolin and add 3 oz. of fruit kernel oil. Remove the pot from the heat and quickly add the 1 oz. of Honeydew juice, beating continually, and add 4–8 drops of compound tincture of Benzoin. The Benzoin is antiseptic and also a natural preservative for the cream which should last in your refrigerator up to a month.

HEALING HOUSELEEK CREAM

Macerate, squeeze, and strain Houseleeks until you have at least 1 oz. of the juice. Melt together 1 oz. lanolin and 3 oz. oil and add the Houseleek juice plus 1 oz. of Fennel water. Add 8 drops of tincture of Benzoin as a preservative. Use the Basic Cream directions.

STIMULATING CIRCULATION LOTION

Steam your skin with a simple mixture of Steaming Herbs. Then apply the following lotion. Make 4 oz. mucilage of Tragacanth using Peppermint water instead of distilled water. Add 1 oz. mucilage of Flax or Quince made with Rosemary/Nettle water. Add 5 drops of tincture of Benzoin and 1 drop of essential oil of Peppermint. Follow the application of the Stimulating Lotion with Peppermint water as a rinse.

EIGHT OILS CLEANSING OIL

There are a number of kinds of oil that can be used for cleansing, and everyone seems to have their own favorites. Mine—a mixture of oils I use in all my creams, lotions, massage or body oils—is as follows: Mix together ½ cup of each of the following oils, shake together completely, put it away, and use it as a base for all your cosmetics requiring oil.

Olive oil	Soy oil
Sesame oil	Fruit kernel oil
Wheat germ oil	Peanut oil
Sunflower oil	Avocado oil

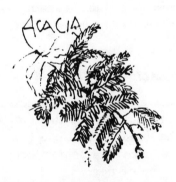

MAYONNAISE CLEANSING CREAM

Beat 1 egg yolk into 4 T. organic health food mayonnaise, 1 t. Carrot seed oil (if you can find it) (or 1 T. Carrot juice), and 1 T. yogurt. Blend together completely and use this at any time of the day for cleansing or moisturizing. Naturally it should be kept in the refrigerator. You could also add a few drops of compound tincture of Benzoin as a natural preservative. This cream is a wonderful skin conditioner and toner. It contains natural vitamin A and lecithin, which is an emulsifying agent capable of attracting moisture to the skin to plump it up and make it look firm.

LEMON CREAM For Oily Skin

4 T. softened Coconut oil
2 T. Witch Hazel extract or boric acid solution
2 T. freshly squeezed and strained Lemon juice

Blend together completely in the mini-blend container of your blender, and put in a jar.

STRAWBERRY CREAM For Oily Skin

1 oz. Strawberry juice
1 oz. Cocoa butter
4 oz. Soy oil

Melt the Cocoa butter in the top of a double boiler, add the Soy oil, and beat together, remove the pot from heat and add the Strawberry juice, beating the mixture until it cools. Add 5 drops of tincture of Benzoin and beat until cold. Follow use with a refreshing rinse of Strawberry water.

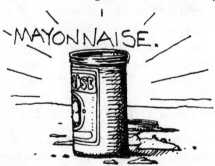

HONEYSUCKLE WRINKLE CREAM

1. Infuse 1 oz. freshly picked Honeysuckle flowers in

5 oz. of nondrying oil for 2 days. Put it in the sun in the daytime and take it in at night.

2. Peel the bark from the Honeysuckle vines until you have a good-sized handful. Soak the bark in 2 cups of water for at least 1 day.

3. Simmer the bark and water for at least 20 minutes. Strain out the bark and simmer the solution down to ½ cup.

4. Add 4 oz. of the strained Honeysuckle flower oil to the bark water and simmer until most of the water has boiled off.

5. Add 1½ oz. solidifier such as lanolin.

6. When everything is melted and incorporated remove from the fire and beat until it is cool.

7. Add some pure essence of Honeysuckle until you get the desired scent and beat until cold.

8. Apply this oil to your wrinkles several times a day until the desired result is obtained.

CUCUMBER WRINKLE REMOVER

Combine in a blender ¼ cup chopped-up Cucumber, 1 egg white, 2 T. mayonnaise, 2 oz. fruit kernel oil. Apply to the skin in the morning and in the evening. Remove excess with tissues. Before going to bed pierce a vitamin E capsule with a pin, squeeze the contents into your hand, and with a gentle fingertip, massage the vitamin E onto the offending wrinkles and allow the E to spend the night.

#193 *from* THE TOILET OF FLORA

Take oil of violets, and the expressed juice of Mallows, of each an ounce and a half; goose grease and veal marrow, of each a quarter of an ounce; Gum Tragacanth, a drachm and a half [about 1½ t.]; melt the whole over a gentle fire.

If you substitute chicken fat or Crisco for the goose

grease you should be able to make this cream that is very soothing for irritated skin.

ECZEMA CREAM

4 oz. Soybean oil	1 oz. Comfrey root water
1 oz. Aloe gel	1½ oz. Cocoa butter

Follow the Basic Cream directions.

Chapter IX

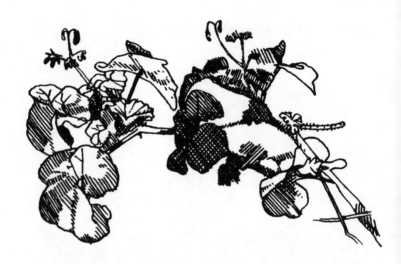

Herbal Masks and Packs
for Every Purpose

Every vegetable, fruit, seed, or nut has a place in a facial or
body mask. Indeed, masks can be used by any sex and any
age of human being and on any part of the body. They are
used to clear up pimples or blackheads, exfoliate the outer
scaly surface of the skin, refine the pores, nourish, heal
and soothe, absorb excess oil, texturize the skin's surface,
moisturize, hydrate, lubricate, or smooth.

FOR DRY TO NORMAL SKIN

Irish Moss   Oranges
Apple   Grapes
Orange Flowers   Avocado
Honeydew Melon   Nectarine
Watermelon   Pears

NORMAL OR AVERAGE SKIN

Tangerine   Crenshaw Melon
Cantaloupe   Banana
Casaba Melon   Citrus
Marigold   Peach
Carrot   Zucchini
Peppermint

NORMAL TO OILY SKIN

Lemongrass   Cherry
Lemon Peel   Lemons
Bananas   Strawberry
Tomato   Apricot Leaves
Persian Melon   Avocado Oil
Peppermint Oil

BASIC FRUIT MASK DIRECTIONS

Facial Masks are used periodically to refine and clean out the pores, to tighten sagging flesh, and to stimulate. After steaming and applying a mask, I feel like my flesh is firmly attached, tight, and slick; it feels good.

1. Mash the fruit.
2. Squeeze out juice.
3. Apply pulp to face.
4. Lie down with legs raised in sun or bath—10 minutes.
5. Rinse off and astringe.

Apples and Pears are used for smoothness. Lemons, Oranges, Grapefruits, and other citrus are tonic and antiseptic. Grapes and Pears are tonic, moisturizing, nourishing, and rejuvenating to the facial muscles. Apricots, Peaches, Nectarines, and Melons refine and texturize the skin. Black Currants and Blueberries are used to protect the skin capillaries; Strawberries and other berries reduce oiliness, are potent degreasers, and make the skin soft like velvet.

ALICE'S HUSBAND'S FAVORITE MASK

Apricot and honey mixed together and applied to a clean moist face are great for skin that has been mistreated by a razor. Apply it while in the shower or bath where the steam can help the honey penetrate. It tastes delicious and can be used on toast if you have any left over after your mask.

SOME COMMON EVERYDAY MASKS

Masks must be applied to a super clean face and they are often more successful after the face has been steam cleaned and/or massaged. We all know about the egg white mask applied to clean skin to stimulate and refine enlarged pores. But have you ever tried beating your egg white into a stiff peak and then applying to the skin? Follow your mask with a rinse of warm, then cool water.

There are natural earth clays such as kaolin, bentonite, and Fuller's earth that have been used as refining masks for years. They are capable of absorbing large quantities of excess oil and are terrific for oily skin with large pores. These clays mixed with mucilage of Tragacanth, Quince, or Seapod gel make the mask soft enough so that it can be removed in one piece.

Cooked Oatmeal or ground-up Oats are also a common ingredient in masks as well as Cornmeal, Buckwheat flour, whole wheat flour, or Almond meal. These flours mixed with any type of milk product such as yogurt or buttermilk are nourishing both for your insides and outsides.

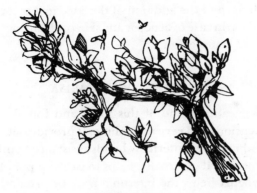

ANY SKIN

The following herbal facial masques are generally useful for any type of skin or combination of skin problems. Always start with a clean, very slightly damp face and neck.

ALOE ALMOND MASQUE For Acne

Mash together some inner pulp from the Aloe plant and some Almond meal—enough to make a small handful. Add some Green Oil (Chapter XXII), or any cold-pressed oil, about 1 tablespoon. Now mix these ingredients together into a nice gooey meal and massage gently into the skin using upward rotating motions. Let it stay on the skin about 10 minutes and then rinse off with warm water. Follow this facial with an astringent—any astringent but particularly Rosewater or Rose Astringent Lotion (see Chapter X).

For a skin tightening mask, I use a bit of warm water or egg white on my hands when mixing this mask instead of the oil. When my face feels too tight or stiff I use the oil. It takes about 20 fresh Almonds, ground to powder in the moulinex mill, and a piece of scraped, peeled Aloe from a leaf about 3½ × 1 × ¼ inch to make enough for 1 generous or 2 skimpy masks. This application is very soothing and refreshing, and the addition of the Aloe makes it a useful application in case of acne, or any skin problem including a too florid complexion.

CARROT YOGURT MASK

We tried eating some of this mask and found it to be quite delicious and very nourishing. It provides vitamin A, which when taken internally builds resistance to infection and, when used externally, helps to clear up pimples and acne; yogurt helps the intestinal tract by promoting the growth of helpful bacteria, and externally, because it is naturally acid balanced, it is neutral on the skin and, in addition, provides natural protein and calcium.

Very slightly cook some Carrots. Take a tablespoon or two of the Carrots and mash thoroughly with some yogurt. Or else you might add some yogurt and a raw scraped Carrot to the miniblend container of a blender and mix for a bit. Now apply the carroty-yogurt to the skin—again with upward rotating movements. Let it stay for a bit and then rinse off with tepid water or a splash of mineral water. If your skin is a bit dry, you can rub the slight residue that is left into the skin or else you can completely remove the mask with a splash of an astringent.

MILK OF ALMONDS MASK

Pound together in a wooden mortar and pestle some Rosewater, honey, and some fresh milky ground-up Almonds (or else Almond meal). Make a paste and apply to a clean face and neck. Scrub about and let it get tacky and dry. Rinse off and apply Rosewater as an astringent.

A student who used this mask liked it very much once it became tacky and could be massaged (masséed) into the skin. When she removed it, she commented that her skin felt very soft and seemed to have tightened up a bit. Honey is an excellent skin tightening, nutritive, and naturally acid-balanced skin food. It is hydrating and since as skin ages it loses moisture, the honey binds up the water and helps the skin to retain rather than lose moisture.

FRESH MINT MASK

Take some fresh Spearmint, chop it up, and mash it fluffy, soft, and green with any cream or oil. Wheat germ oil would be especially nice. Apply it to a nice clean face as an evening application. Let it stay on the face and neck for 15 minutes and then rinse it off. It will leave a very slight oily residue that can be gently massaged into the skin as a night cream; or else apply an astringent.

With too much oil, the Mint will lose its refreshing qualities. This mask is especially useful on middle-aged skin that is a bit dry and tight feeling.

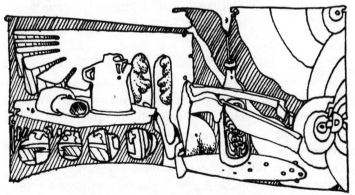

YELLOW EGG YOLK MASH MASK

Mash a raw egg yolk with a bit of oil and 1 t. of powdered Camomile flowers and apply *evenly* on a clean face. Leave it on for about 15 minutes and then rinse with very warm water and apply a bit of honey. Pat it on the skin. Rinse with tepid water and apply an astringent. Terrific, a great pick-me-up and rejuvenator when your poor old face is tired. (See *The International Beauty Book* for a variation of this mask.)

THE SAN CLEMENTE ORANGE

Peel an Orange, skin it, and mash the pulp, or else put the peeled Orange or half an Orange into the blender and blend. Add some yellow Cornmeal and mix until gritty. Apply to the usual clean, slightly moist face. Let it stay for a few minutes or steam with Orange Flower-Orange Peel Mix (Chapter VII). Rinse carefully with tepid water or mineral water. Apply an astringent of Orange Flower water.

This wonderful mask makes the skin feel very fresh and wonderfully clean and is used when fatigued and to prevent aging. San Clemente reminds my husband of hot supermarkets and parking lots; so when your feet are hot and your eyeballs feel like they are falling out of your face from the heat apply the San Clemente Orange.

THE HONEY PAT

The Honey Pat mask is just about the most useful and all-around perfect creation made by nature. It can be used by everyone. When I first started experimenting with natural cosmetics and organic beautifiers, I usually performed these interesting ablutions in the bathtub out of sight of my family. My family, as most, thinks that mother in the bathtub with a ring of herbs around her or with sticky gooey stuff on the face is really a delight, a humorous thing to be commented on and laughed about. But they all like to use the Honey Pat.

Dip your fingers into a bit of honey and apply it to your

face in an upward revolving motion. Now pat your face with your fingertips as if you were typing a letter on your face. It will soon get so tacky that you can barely pull your fingers away. *Stop* typing. Rinse your face with tepid water or mineral water. Honey is a natural rejuvenator and humectant and leaves you feeling refreshed and invigorated. Skin ages not because it loses its ability to hold oil, but because it loses its ability to retain moisture. Honey is a natural hydrater, that is, it seems to have the capacity to maintain or restore the normal proportion of water in the skin. The Honey Pat feels smooth and leaves the skin lightly tight and firm with a warm feeling and light, pleasant smell. Because the honey is acid, it helps to rid the face of blemishes and blackheads.

THE MONSTER MASK

Yech! Horrible to look at but a delight to experience and positively one of the most soothing, smoothing treats for dry or normal skin, especially those troubled with dry flaky patches.

Cook up a small batch of old-fashioned Oatmeal. The gooey sticky kind. While the Oatmeal is cooking, pour ½ cup of boiling water over about 4 dried Prunes that are in a small pot. When the Oatmeal is cooked and the Prunes are soft, mash up a bit of Prune with a bit of Oatmeal, blend all together really well with a ripe juicy Fig in a mini-blender or with a wooden spoon. Now would be a good time to take a soaky bath, adding all that extra colloidal Oatmeal that you made, or you can eat the Oatmeal for breakfast with some honey: it's quite delicious. Then apply the Fig, Prune and Oatmeal mess, also called the Monster Mask—to your face, jump into your tub, let the mask dry as much as it will and then rinse it all off and pat your skin dry. This mask is a natural laxative and flushes all the nasties right out of the pores. It might be a good idea to precede the Monster Mask with a cleansing herbal facial steam.

DRY SKIN MASKS

ADAM AND EVE'S FAVORITE MASK

Warm, freshly made Applesauce, mixed with a bit of wheat germ to make a paste and applied to a warm dry face, is a splendid mixture for dry skin. The Applesauce mixed with cooked Oatmeal is very soothing for windburned or sunburned skin.

GREEN GOO

Chop up some Parsley and blend it in a blender with a little bit of honey and a drop or two of chlorophyll. It should be thick enough to make a thick paste. Apply to your face with rotating upward and outward movements of the fingertips. Leave the mask on your skin to harden as much as it will for at least 20 minutes. Then rinse off with warm water or steam it for a minute or two. Finally rinse with cool water or a flower water.

ESPECIALLY FOR IRRITATED OR DELICATE SKIN

Mix equal quantities of powdered Comfrey root, powdered Irish Moss, and enough glycerin to make a paste. Apply this and let it stay on your face while you shower or bathe, then wash off, and follow it with a rinse of fresh skim milk.

THE CALIFORNIA AVOCADO

Mash a bit of Avocado with a bit of buttermilk and apply directly to the face. Walk around or lie in the sun and let the Avocado with its nourishing oils do the work. Wipe off the excess with soft tissues and rinse with tepid water. Now, gently massage the invisible oily remains into your skin.

CACTUS MASK

Mix together an equal quantity of *Aloe vera* gel and Grape pulp and apply to the face. Precede with a steam for dry skin and follow it with a light application of Quince seed gel.

EARTH MASK FOR REFINING PORES

Mix clay or Fuller's earth and powdered Dulse with egg white or Seaweed gel to a paste and apply to clean damp skin. Let it harden, remove, and rinse with warm, then cool, water. Add enough Seaweed gel and it will remove in one piece, taking the impurities with it.

OILY SKIN MASKS

BREWER'S YEAST AND LEMON GRASS

Brewer's yeast is highly stimulating and should not be used on delicate or highly sensitive skin. But it is terrific on

oily skin. Mix a bit of Brewer's yeast with powdered Lemongrass and yogurt. Apply to clean dry skin and let it stay until hardened. Rinse with warm water and apply a soothing moisturizer such as Aloe gel or mucilage of Quince.

MASHED TOMATO MASK

Peel and deseed a Tomato, using only the firm pulp for your mask. Mash the pulp and mix with enough Oatmeal to make a thick but smooth paste. Apply to your skin.

DICK'S FAVORITE MASK For Oily Skin

Dick's skin is very oily-looking and covered with blemishes; he thinks this mask makes his face feel clean and alive, and we know it makes him look 100 per cent more handsome. First steam with any facial herb mixture, then mix a mask of powdered Comfrey root, powdered Apricot, ground Oats, and powdered Lemongrass. It is cooling and mildly astringent. Remove your mask with warm water and follow with a splash of the liquid left from the herbal steaming.

LEMON AND CUCUMBER

Mash some Cucumber in a mortar, add some Lemon juice and enough Almond meal to make a paste. This is mildly astringent and yet soothing.

Chapter X

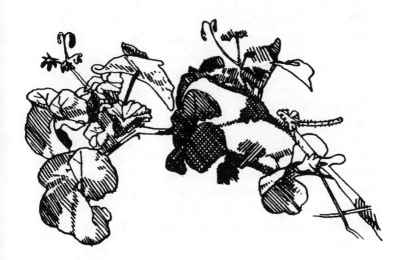

Herbal Astringents, Cosmetic Vinegars, Facial Waters, and Aftershave

A STILL is required to make really perfect Facial Waters and Aftershave Lotions. You can go to a laboratory supply house and get expensive exotic glassware and corks or you can poke around your neighborhood and in your kitchen and manufacture a homemade still at home.

A SIMPLE STILL

Get a container that can be sealed, about 1½ to 2 gallons in size. Enamel ware, stainless steel, tin, or glassware will do; it should have a large neck. This container is now called the retort or cucurbit. Fit a cork that has had a ½-inch-wide hole drilled into it, tightly into the neck. Fit tightly into this hole ½-inch-wide glass or tin tubing about 4 feet long. The tubing should be bent into an elongated, upside-down U-shape, passing into the neck of a second container of like size (now called the receiver), and going down into the receiver about two-thirds of the way. The receiver should be wrapped in wetted wool or heavy flannel in order for it to be kept cool and condense the steam. It is then set in a shallow pan containing some water, but not enough to make the receiver unsteady. Put a layer of clean stones in the bottom of the cucurbit to keep the plants from being burned, fill it loosely with the substance you wish to distill (alternately, you could put a plate or sieve in the bottom of the cucurbit to put the plants on), add about a gallon of water, and put it on the fire to boil. The water will boil, the steam will pass from the cucurbit through the tubing to be

flat salt flints still flints salts flats still

condensed into liquid in the receiver. Stop when you have about a half gallon of liquid (Flower or Facial Water) in the receiver.

A SIMPLE STILL FOR DISTILLING FACIAL AND FLOWER WATER

Take a deep glass or enamel pot with a rounded top. Center a rack in the bottom of the pot to hold a smaller enamel bowl off the bottom. The bigger pot is the cucurbit and the smaller the receiver. Put enough botanical substance in the bottom of the larger pot to come halfway up the smaller bowl and add hot water to just cover the botanicals. Put the rounded lid in upside down, and fill this upside down lid with ice and icy water. Put this contraption on the fire. The water boils, the steam rises, hits the ice cold lid, condenses and drips into the bowl in the center of the pot. You should probably have an ice cube or two (made from distilled water) in the smaller enamel bowl to start the process.

A SIMPLE TEAPOT STILL

Fill a teapot loosely with herbs or flowers (cucurbit), add enough water to cover the botanical material, attach enough rubber tubing to the spout so that the center part can rest in a pan of ice water and empty into a small bowl (receiver) about a foot away from the teapot. Bring the teapot to a boil, turn the fire to low and simmer until at least half of the water has boiled off. The water boils, the steam comes out of the spout, condenses in the ice water bath, and is collected in the receiver as Flower Water.

CERTAIN METHODS TO IMPROVE THE COMPLEXION

Brown ladies should frequently bathe themselves, and wash their faces with a few drops of Spirit of Wine, sometimes with Virgin's Milk, and the distilled Waters of Pimpernel, White Tansy, Bean Fowers, &c. These detersive penetrating applications, by degrees remove the kind of varnish that covers the skin, and thus render more free the perspiration, which is the only real cosmetic.

—#260, *The Toilet of Flora*

HOW TO MAKE COSMETIC WATER WITHOUT A STILL

When you wish to make a facial water of green herbs or seeds, macerate with a mortar and pestle or bruise with the back of a wooden spoon, about 1 oz. herbs in about 1 cup of water. Put this into a small nonmetal pot, add 1 more cup of water, cover, bring to a low boil and *simmer* for a few minutes. Turn the heat off and let it infuse until cool. Strain carefully into a clean bottle through muslin or cheesecloth and store in the refrigerator. Use the strained herbs as compost in your garden. This water will spoil —unlike distilled waters which will last for months—so make only enough to last a few days. If you wish to preserve the water for a little longer, add ¼ oz. or less tincture of Benzoin to 1 cup of cosmetic water. Shake thoroughly before each use; the added tincture of Benzoin will turn the solution milky.

If you wish to make a facial water of flowers or other delicate materials, put 1 oz. fresh or dried flowers in a small nonmetal pot and add 1 cup of water, preferably distilled water. Bruise the flowers gently with the back of a wooden spoon, and add 1 more cup of water. Either heat ever so gently on the stove for a few minutes or put the pot in the sun and let the sun heat it for a few hours. Strain through absolutely clean cheesecloth (use the strained flowers as mulch for house plants), store in a clean bottle, refrigerate, and use as an after-washing rinse whenever necessary. This will also spoil, so make only enough for a few days at a time. Add ⅛ oz. tincture of Benzoin to 1 cup of the Flower Water for added protection against blemishes and as a natural preservative. This type of solution was originally called Virgin's Milk as it turned milky when shaken.

A COOLING WASH

Infuse in a sufficient quantity of clear Water, some Bran, Yolks of Eggs, and a grain or two of Ambergrise, for three or four hours; then distil the Water, which will prove an excellent Cosmetic, and clear the skin surprisingly. It is of service to keep it in the sun eight or ten days, in a bottle well corked.

The distilled Waters of Melons, Bean Flowers, the Wild-Vine, green or unripe Barley, and the Water that is found is vesicles on the leaves of the elm-tree may also be used for the same intention.

—*The Toilet of Flora,* 1779

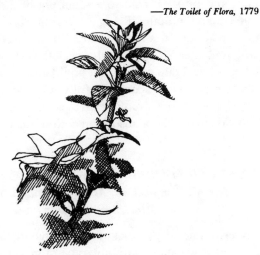

TO CLEAR A BABY'S FACE OF PIMPLES

. . . Skin kept white and cleere. Wash the face and body of a sucking childe with breast milke, or cow milk, or mixed with water, every night: and the child's skin will wax fair and cleere, and resist Sun burning.

—*Delightes for Ladies*, 1602

AN EXCELLENT HAND WATER OR WASHING WATER VERY CHEAPE

Take a gallon of faire water, one handful of Lavender flowers, a few Cloves and some Orris powder, and four ounces of Beniamin (benzoin): distill the water in an ordinarie leaden Still. You may distill a second water by a new infusion of water upon the seces: a little of this will sweeten a bason of faire water for your table.

—*Delightes for Ladies*, 1602

COOLING SKIN WATER FOR RED OR FLUSHED FACES

Take a handful, about 1 ounce, of freshly picked Peppermint and infuse it cold in a small pot in 2 cups distilled water for a few hours. Bring it to a gentle boil and *simmer* it ever so gently for a few minutes. Strain carefully through absolutely clean, extra fine cheesecloth and cool. Dissolve 1 t. Sea salt in 1 cup of the Mint liquid and bring it to a boil, skimming off any scum carefully. Cool and refrigerate. This is a wonderful application to acne or scabby pimples; dab it on with a bit of absorbent cotton. Also very stimulating.

THAT OLD STANDBY * ROSEWATER & GLYCERIN * For All Complexions, As an Aftershave, a Soothing Rinse After Washing

Glycerin is now a product of the petroleum industry. You can make this lotion with any type of glycerin, but if you can find pure old-fashioned glycerin, that is what you should use. Glycerin is a natural moisturizer and Rosewater, a mild and pleasant astringent. The combination is perfect for everyone except the unfortunate few who may be allergic to glycerin. Start with your own homemade distilled Rosewater or go to the nearest chemist, liquor store, or pharmacy and buy triple distilled Rosewater. Now you're ready. There are many versions of glycerin and Rosewater. Make up your own recipe or use one of the following:

4 oz. glycerin:	4 oz. Rosewater	
4 T. glycerin:	4 oz. Rosewater:	4 T. mucilage of Tragacanth
4 oz. glycerin: for oily skin	4 oz. Rosewater:	1 t. Lemon juice
4 oz. glycerin: for dry skin	4 oz. Rosewater:	1 t. pure honey
2 oz. glycerin: lotion	4 oz. Rosewater:	2 oz. cornhuskers

Shake together and store in a small lightproof container in a cool dark place.

LOTION FOR CHAPS

2 t. borax   4 oz. glycerin
12 oz. triple Rosewater   3 T. mucilage of Quince

Mix together.

CUCUMBER ANTIWRINKLE LOTION

Cucumbers contain a useful antiwrinkle hormone and their pH is about 5.5 which is the same as healthy skin. Wash and scrub a Cucumber. Slice it and mash it well with a mortar and pestle. Add ¼ cup Rosewater and macerate the cuke. Strain carefully through clean cheesecloth. Melt about 1 T. anhydrous lanolin, add 2 oz. Comfrey root water and beat until cold. Add the Cucumber-Rosewater and beat until incorporated. You could also add one 500-unit capsule of vitamin E for every ½ oz. of liquid.

EVER WONDER WHY MEN HAVE LESS WRINKLES?

Because they shave them off every day that they shave. Shaving removes the outer layer of the skin, and instead of wrinkle lotion around the mouth, they need a skin soothing tonic.

Mix together 2 oz. Witch Hazel extract, 2 oz. mucilage of Quince, and a few drops of either Lemon oil or Peppermint oil to scent it.

A COSMETIC WATER

Excellent as an eye wash, mildly astringent, makes a cooling and nourishing wash for the skin and the mouth. Wash the face with the tears that issue from the Vine, during the months of May and June.

—*The Toilet of Flora,* 1779

AN EXCELLENT COSMETIC

Pimpernel Water is so sovereign a beautifier of the complexion, that it ought always to have a place on a Lady's toilet.

—*The Toilet of Flora,* 1779

LAVENDER WATER

Freshly made every few days, Lavender Water is delightful as an aftershave lotion for men's faces or ladies' legs. It is mildly astringent, nonalcoholic, aromatic, reduces puffiness, and is useful as a topical application for acne.

FACIAL WATER For Oily Skin

Mix together equal quantities of Comfrey root, Witch Hazel bark, and Fennel seed, enough to make 1 ounce. Macerate with the back of a wooden spoon in a small nonmetal pot with 2 cups of water. Cover the pot and infuse for an hour, *simmer* for 20 minutes, and infuse until cold. Strain and refrigerate the water. Comfrey root is great as a mulch for all kinds of plants, so use the strained herbs in your garden or on house plants as organic nourishment for them.

WITCH HAZEL EXTRACT

This extract is great by itself or mixed half and half with Rosewater, for bruises, bug bites, to cool a sunburn, as a compress for scalds and burns, aftershave lotion, mouthwash, as a rub for muscle aches, as a footbath for sore, tired and burning feet, and as a hair rinse after shampooing.

FACIAL WATER For Dry or Puffy Skin

Mix together Camomile and Fennel, enough of each to make 1 ounce. Add 1 cup of water and macerate the whole with the back of a wooden spoon. Infuse cold for 20 minutes and then heat gently for 10 more. Cool and strain through silk. This mixture is delicate enough for the most sensitive skin; I use it as a wash for my baby's fair white body.

MILK AND HONEY For Aging Skin

Heat gently in an 8 oz. enamel cup, 1 oz. of Orange Honey. Remove from heat. Add 6 oz. of raw skim milk. Mix together completely, and use this as a rinse by patting it on with cotton balls night and morning.

BRACING SKIN TONIC

Any of the melons or fruits used fresh and raw make excellent nourishing, refreshing skin tonics. After you wash your face, take a slice of your morning fruit and pat it briskly all over your face and neck; then, pat dry with a hand towel. Apples, Honeydew Melons, and Pears can be used for dry skin. Grapes, Oranges, and Cantaloupes can be used for average skin, and Lemons, Tomatoes, Straw-berries, and Persian Melons can be used for oily skin.

Other Facial Waters can be made from any of the herbs: Yarrow for astringency and oily skin; Sage and Sagebrush for men as aftershave lotions; Camomile for dry skin; Peppermint, which contains menthol, as a cooling, stimulating lotion for hot sunny days; and Camphor for pimples.

COSMETIC AND FACIAL VINEGARS

The same herbs that you would use in facial waters are also used in the vinegars. They are easy to make, and the vinegar preserves the botanical essences and so can be stored for periods of time. All you have to do is heat 2 cups of vinegar to the boiling point and add 1 oz. of herb, bottle and infuse for 10 days, shake the bottle daily, strain and use. Apple cider vinegar is preferred but you can also use plain white vinegar. When you wish to use the vinegar, dilute it by half with water or Rosewater and use as a facial rinse, vaginal douche, mouthwash, aftershave lotion, or salad dressing. It is softening and will relieve itchy skin and restore the natural acid balance. Check Chapters I and III for the herbs to use. Combinations such as Comfrey, Licorice, and Camomile or Comfrey, Lavender, Rose-mary, and Sage are equally potent.

ROSE ASTRINGENT LOTION

Bring to a boil 3 cups of white vinegar, remove to a bottle, and add ½ oz. Rosebuds, ¼ oz. Myrtle berries, ¼ oz. Camomile flowers, and ½ oz. Jamaica flowers. Infuse the botanicals for 10 days and shake the bottle daily. Strain carefully through cheesecloth and add an equal quantity of Rosewater. This makes an absolutely delightful facial lotion, aftershave lotion, or underarm deodorant. Really terrific!

SAGE AFTERSHAVE LOTION

Infuse ½ oz. Sage and Rosemary combined in 1 cup of Apple cider vinegar for a week. Strain. Add an equal quantity of Witch Hazel extract.

GERANIUM LOTION

Infuse ½ oz. assorted scented Geranium leaves in 1 cup of vinegar for 5–10 days. Strain and use as a stimulating, refreshing astringent. Dilute with water to use.

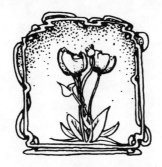

AMBER'S SUPER DUPER
EXTRA SPECIAL DYNAMITE
COSMETIC VINEGAR AND REFRESHER

Take 1 oz. of each of the following herbs: Spearmint, Pansy leaf, Comfrey root, Rosemary, Lavender, Elder flowers, Myrtle leaf, Orange peel, Camomile flowers, and Basil. Bruise them and infuse in 1½ quarts of fine quality vinegar that has been brought to a boil. Shake this mixture daily for 10 days. In the meantime in a smaller bottle put ½ oz. gum Camphor, ¼ oz. macerated Clove buds, ½ oz. Myrrh gum, ¼ oz. gum Benzoin, and add 4 oz. tincture of Benzoin. Shake this mixture daily for 10 days and strain through coarse cheesecloth. At the end of the 10 days, strain the vinegar mixture through another piece of cheesecloth, mix the two liquids together and shake them daily for 3 days. At the end of 3 days, strain the final mixture through another piece of cheesecloth into an amber bottle. This fine cosmetic vinegar is used by adding a *few drops* of it to a cup of water as a rinse for the face. It is energizing and stimulating, restoring the natural acid balance to the skin; it is cooling and soothing and can be added to the bath or to the shower. It will ease itchy skin and sunburn, relieve a tired body when used in the bath, and is a stimulating foot bath. I use about an ounce at a time in my bathtub and a teaspoonful in the baby's bath.

Chapter XI

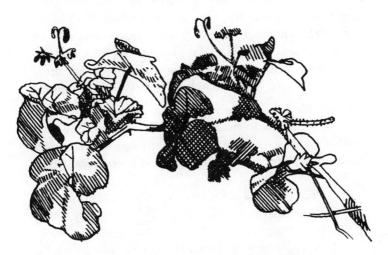

Homemade Soaps
for Every Purpose

To soap or not to soap. Most dermatologists say that claims made about soap being harmful and drying to the skin are grossly exaggerated. Soap and water washing is deliciously refreshing; soap's alkalinity is one of the factors that enable it to clean so efficiently. Dr. Erno Laszlo was one of the proponents of twice a day soap and water washing. I believe he is the one who said something like, "A skin washed with cream can never be clean." So the question is not should you or should you not wash with soap, but what soap should you wash with that best suits your skin type, and how often should you use it?

You can buy all sorts of soaps at your local pharmacy, department store, or specialty store. I personally have used over 300 different kinds of soap. Some of the better soap outlets in the United States include the Soap Opera in Madison, Wisconsin; Caswell-Massey in New York City; and Truc International, Inc. in Woodstock Hill, Connecticut. Truc wholesales and distributes soaps from all over the world, and they have been kind enough to send me dozens of samples to try out. I must say that the last three years of the soap experiment have been most interesting.[1]

Homemade Soap is really quite easy to make. In *Herbs & Things,* complete directions on how to make your own high quality castile soap are given. Basically you will want a fat solution at 125° to be slowly mixed into a lye solution at 90°.

1. Add 6 cups of water to 13 oz. of lye and cool to 90°.
2. Now add the lye solution to 6 lb. of fat (5 lb. of clean fat or lard and 1 lb. of Olive oil) that is at 125°.
3. Stir steadily until this mixture is thick and creamy. It may take an hour.
4. Add scent if you like.
5. Pour into greased molds or into a cloth-lined wet wooden box.
6. Let the soap dry for awhile—4 hours to a week.
7. Unmold it or cut it into bars and then let it age for at least a month.

This is an extremely simplistic description of what soapmaking is all about but if you will write: Pennwalt Corporation, Product Information, 3 Parkway, Philadelphia, Pennsylvania 19102, they will send you more complete soapmaking directions. Ask for their pamphlet called

[1]My new book in progress, *The Herbal Soap Book,* is an entire book on the 300 different soaps that I have made, purchased and used.

"Notes on Soapmaking." You can also ask for CA-72-35 from the USDA, Agricultural Research Service, Southern Marketing and Nutrition Research Division, New Orleans, Louisiana 70119; it's called "Soap Making at Home."

Once you have your castile soap whether store-bought or homemade, you can make all sorts of wonderful made-to-order-to-your-personal-skin-type of soap. You can buy castile soap by the slab at many, many fine stores around the world including Caswell-Massey in New York and Conti soaplets from Indiana Botanic in Hammond, Indiana.

JELLIED CAMOMILE SOAP For Washing Faces and Delicate Lingerie

Bring to a boil 6 cups of water and 2–3 oz. of Camomile flowers. Simmer gently for 20 minutes, take off the heat, and infuse until cool. In the meantime shred pure mild hand soap or castile soap until you have 2 cups. Strain out the flowers and bring 3 cups of the Camomile water to a boil, add the soap and ½ cup of borax. Stir and boil for a few minutes and then remove from the heat and let the soap cool. It will form a jelly-like consistency. Pour it into containers and keep covered. Obviously you can substitute any herb for the Camomile, say Lemongrass for oily skin, Comfrey root and Marshmallow flowers or Carrots for dry skin, Peppermint for aromatic astringency, Yarrow plus a scent for an astringent soap, Lavender to wash lingerie, etc. You can also add scent to the solution, ¼ oz. The consistency of this soap depends on two things: the kind of castile soap you start with and the herb you use. Since different manufacturers use different formulations for castile soap it follows that the quantity of water to soap will vary. The harder the soap the more water is needed to soften it. The type I use requires only about 2 cups of herbed water to 2 cups of shaved soap. Also when I use mucilaginous herbs like Comfrey root and Marshmallow root, it requires more like 3 cups herbed water to 2 cups soap. So play around with the amounts to come up with the consistency you like best.

HONEY SOAP For Burns and Scalds and Sensitive Skin

Mix and melt together, 4 oz. of shaved white soap, 4 oz. of honey, 1 oz. Pimpernel or Houseleek or Comfrey water. This soap is very soothing.

A SOAP TO TAKE OUT ALL KINDS OF STAINS

Boil a handful of strawberries or Strawberry leaves in a quart of Water and a pint of Vinegar, adding two pounds of Castile Soap, and half a pound of Chalk in fine powder; boil them together till the water has evaporated. When you use it wet the place with the sharpest Vinegar or Verjuice, and rub it over with this Soap; dry it afterwards before the fire or in the Sun.

—*The Toilet of Flora*, 1779

CLEANSING CORNMEAL SOAP

Cornmeal soap is great as an invigorating cleanser. I like to use it after a strenuous workout at the spa. In the top of a double boiler, put 1 cup Corn juice or plain water and 1 lb. shaved castile soap. When the soap is melted stir in ½ lb. Cornmeal, more or less, depending on the grittiness you like. Let it cool enough until you can work it by hand. Grease your hand and work the soap into balls; then store away for use.

ALMOND MEAL SOAP

This soap is gritty and has a slight bleaching action. It is made as above but use Almond milk or Comfrey water in place of the Corn juice. Use ½ lb. of Almond meal to 1 lb. of shaved soap.

TAR SOAP For Eczema and Psoriasis

Take about 1 lb. of castile soap and melt it with 'a little water. When it is melted but thick add up to 1½ oz. of wood tar[1]. Stir and beat it thoroughly to prevent lumps. Mold by hand or cut into cakes.

LANOLIN SOAP IS LUBRICATING AND GOOD
For Dry Skin

In one pot melt 1 lb. of shaved castile soap with 1 cup of Comfrey root or Parsley water. In another pot gently melt 1–4 oz. of anhydrous lanolin. When the two are melted, add the lanolin slowly into the soap, stirring continually until well blended. Cool and cut into cakes.

HERBAL SOAPS OF LETTUCE, CUCUMBER, STRAWBERRIES, OR CARROTS

Cut 4 oz. of the botanical into pieces, macerate it in 1 cup of water with the back of a wooden spoon, *simmer* in the top of a double boiler for 10 minutes. Infuse until cool, strain through cheesecloth removing any particles. Take the resulting liquid and pour into 4–16 oz. of shaved castile soap (depends on how solid a piece of soap you want), and heat until the soap is melted and the juices are well incorporated. Let it cool, add appropriate scents if you like, and cut into bars.

[1]Wood tar is available from Indiana Botanic and Homoeopathic Pharmacies.

Scenting Soaps can be difficult because flower scents seem to get lost in the soap, and herb scents are oftentimes irritating to the skin. Bergamot oil is often irritating, but try Sage oil when making Lettuce soap, Strawberry essence for Strawberry soap. Rosemary and Lavender oil are also nice, as well as the citrus oils, Lemon, Grapefruit, Orange, and Lime.

COMFREY ALOE JELLY SOAP
For Sensitive, Irritated or Dry Skin

Make a thick jellied soap using Comfrey root water: Bring to a boil 6 cups water, 2 oz. Comfrey root-CS, and 1 oz. Comfrey leaf-CS. Simmer gently for 20 minutes, take off the heat and infuse until cool. In the meantime, shred pure mild hand soap or castile soap until you have 2 cups. Strain out the Comfrey (mulch your plants with it) and bring 3 cups of the Comfrey water to a low boil, add the 2 cups of soap, stir until dissolved, and remove from the heat. Take about 1 cup of the hot soap and add up to ½ cup Aloe gel (the clear jelly from inside the leaves). Stir with a fork or blend on low speed in a blender until thoroughly incorporated. Store the Aloe Jelly Soap covered until needed. Store the rest of the Comfrey Jelly Soap away in your fridge, covered, until you need it.

ABRASIVE SOAP For Dirty or Greasy Hands

Take ½ lb. of your shaved castile soap and dissolve it in 1 cup of water. (Comfrey or Houseleek water would be good here as it is soothing and healing.) Add 1–2 T. of vegetable oil and work it in completely. Add ½ to 1 lb. of powdered pumice stone (available from pharmacies, such as Nature's Herb Co. in California), and incorporate until well blended and free from lumps. Add up to 1 oz. of Rosemary oil, cover tightly, and store away for use.

A SELECTED ASSORTMENT OF SOME SPECIAL STORE-BOUGHT HERBAL SOAPS[1]

Almond Milk soap from Italy, available through Truc and many fine stores, smells marvelously fresh and was used by Eric when he had a rash on his bottom. It was nonirritating and nondrying and lasted through 14 long soaky baths.

Black Forest Aromatic soap, made in West Germany by Bergmann and Co., distributed by Truc and available wherever I have looked, is an absolutely terrific combination of extracts of Lavender, Thyme, Sage, and Pine, and oils of Arnica, St. Johnswort, Rosemary, and Spike lavender with various mosses. As my mother always said, "Dynamo"! This soap is one of our all-time favorites and smells absolutely delightful on the skin.

Puhls in Germany makes many wonderful soaps. One that we like especially well is **Carnation.**

Doney jabon de Tocador from Barcelona, Spain, available at Caswell-Massey. It is made of marine algae, has a texture like Oatmeal, and is wonderful as a gritty, scrubbing type of soap.

Herbal Potpourri soap made by Abenin of Berlin and available through Truc, is made from Horsetail, Yarrow, Witch hazel, and Camomile. It's best for oily skin, and is relatively inexpensive.

F. Wolff & Sohn in Baden makes some of the most delightful and delicious soaps that I have ever used. The scent is terrific and the quality perfect. I particularly like the Carnation soap (**Nelke**) and the **Indische Blumen Seife.** Truc carries most of the Wolff & Sohn soaps.

---

[1]The addresses of these stores are in Chapter VI.

Neca 7, Lavender-scented, is super, absolutely terrific. It leaves your skin smelling delicious. This soap (it's not really soap because it is made through the wonders of chemistry) is made in Israel, has a neutral pH, and is perfect for sensitive, delicate skin. It is recommended by dermatologists and pediatricians, and I use it on my little boy almost daily. I can easily say this is our favorite soap. It is distributed by Truc and is available through many fine specialty stores.

Neutrogena (made with pure tallow and good enough to eat) and **Savon Clair** are two of the best neutral glycerin-type soaps I know of.

Nova Oatmeal soap made by McCormack's of Dun Laoghaire, Ireland, and available through Truc is used by Mike and helped to ease the itch of his Herpes. It is very long-lasting, is made from edible Oatmeal in a superfatted castile soap base. Terrific!

Original Finnish Sauna soap, made in Finland, available through Truc, is extremely long lasting and wonderfully refreshing.

Royal Jelly soap made in England and available through Truc. This is what Debbie says, "It was so smooth and it slithered between the folds of my body, I noticed how milky white the water became, my skin has once again begun to squeak and the evolution of body odor can begin once again."

Sinalca soap, pH 7, made in Switzerland and available through Caswell-Massey among other places, is made from Swiss milk and wheat germ oil. Really nice.

Spring Glory, made in Spain, available through Caswell-Massey, is made from beeswax and honey to nourish and clean the skin. One of our favorites.

Pure Swiss Buttermilk soap, available through Truc, is a wonderful soap with a delicate smell and especially effective on smog-choked skin. This is one of my choices as a traveling soap (for places like New York and Los Angeles).

Wright's Coal Tar soap made in England is wonderful for skin blemishes and problems like eczema and acne.

Crabtree & Evelyn in England makes many wonderful soaps. We particularly like **Maise Meal soap** (Cornmeal). Very cleansing, slightly abrasive, is useful as an invigorating wake-up soap.

This is only a very brief selection of the number of types of wonderful soaps available in the world. There must be thousands of others. In the United States we like **Ivory** best.

Chapter XII

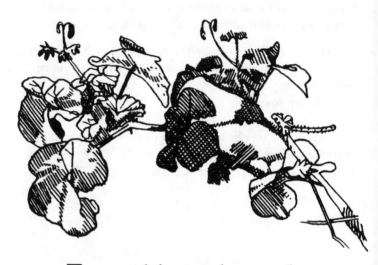

Everything above the Collarbone: Eyes, Nose, Mouth, Teeth, Ears, and Throat

Do YOUR *eyebrows* stick up, act unruly, and need shine? Make a little southernwood oil and use it twice a day as a gloss and strengthener. You can also use this oil to stimulate your *eyelashes* to grow thick and long. But put the oil only on the eyelash and not the eyelids. Try applying it with a cotton-wrapped toothpick. A long-standing folk remedy to stimulate eyelashes to grow is to rub them daily with castor oil or olive oil and use a thick decoction of Sage to darken them and make them less unruly.

Ice cold milk is used in many ways in herbal cosmetics, as an ingredient in more complicated formulas and also by itself. Lie down, dip cotton balls in icy milk and apply the balls to *swollen eyelids*. For *tired eyes, red eyes, puffy eyes* try different herbal concoctions. Some of the best are: for toning, a compress of Comfrey leaf followed by a vitamin E eye pat; for refreshing, soak Cucumber slices in fresh raw milk, lie down, and apply the slices to your eyes; to reduce puffiness, make some ordinary tea extra strong, refrigerate it (add honey if you like), chill the tea bags, and apply them as a compress and drink the tea, the tannin in the tea is nicely astringent; for reducing bags and dark circles try a thin slice of Casaba Melon or Pear under each eye while taking a 10 minute rest, or juice some Parsley in a juicer, add a teaspoon of instant Ginseng to a tablespoon of the Parsley and a bit of mucilage or jello to hold it together and apply this to the eye area while taking a rest. Do it whenever and how often you deem necessary; *puffy eyes* can also be greatly helped by raising the head of your bed a few inches off the floor; this prevents excess body fluid from accumulating in the loose tissue around the eye. Sleep on your back with a small pillow only under the neck and start your mornings with a compress of milk, tea, Lavender, or Cucumber. For *watering eyes,* wash them often with decoctions of Fennel roots, Parsley, Betony, Comfrey root or leaves, honey and Rue or Chervil. Fennel seed water is also good for *tired eyes* as a compress, wash, or drops. For nourishing *tired eyes* try Apple compress; fresh raw sliced Potatoes are terrific for *circles* and *bags*. Whenever using herbal remedies, do make and use your ingredients as quickly as possible; it wouldn't be good at all to introduce any infection where there had been none before by using herbal waters made the day before yesterday. So make Fennel seed water now and use it now or, at best, refrigerate it only overnight. *Eyes* are also benefited by a decoction of Golden Seal and Eyebright as an eyewash or compress.

As for those store-bought eye creams that cost a fortune, the very finest are made at home. Formulate an eye cream for that fragile thin skin around the eye. Try

SUPER EMOLLIENT CREAM

1 oz. lanolin

½ oz Almond oil

½ oz. Apricot kernel oil

enough vitamin E capsules to supply 2500 units/oz.

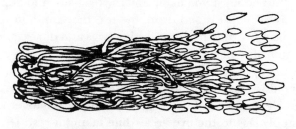

Melt the lanolin in a tiny pan, add the oils and put up in a tiny jar. Gently massage this cream into the area around the eyes to reduce those lines and wrinkles. Remember that persistence will pay off here, so don't give up after a week has elapsed saying that it didn't work for you. If you are lazy, pierce a vitamin E capsule and use the oil directly on the wrinkles.

For *sty in the eye,* wash with California poppy water or warm buttermilk or very weak salted water.

Tiny *broken veins* or *thread veins* will respond well to various herbs. There is absolutely no substitute for good food, rest, and exercise for encouraging a handsome complexion, so first increase vitamins P (permeability) and C; eat and drink lots of Violet leaf tea plus Orange peel (Violet leaf contains more C than Oranges), and then, when you eat the Oranges, eat the white part under the skin also. Compresses of Marigolds, Coltsfoot, Witch Hazel, Parsley, Arnica, and Comfrey work well, especially combinations of these herbs such as Marigold and Comfrey or Parsley juice and Violet leaves. Use these latter combinations both inside as a tea and outside as a compress.

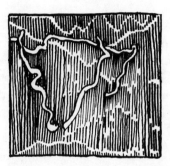

Your *nose* is often neglected and usually has enlarged dirty pores around the nostrils. Make an egg white mask with a drop or two of Lemon juice to tighten the pores of the nose and degrease the oily areas on the face. Naturally you will start with a facial steam or at least a clean face. Apply the egg white/Lemon juice with a small clean paint brush and let the mask dry on the nose. Rinse with warm water, then splash with seltzer or mineral water and pat dry. You can also use the gritty insides of an Avocado peel as a cleansing exfoliant. The water from boiled Lemon and Orange peels is useful for a **red nose.**

Freckles and blemishes are considerably diminished with a Horseradish-buttermilk wash. Just grate 1 T. of Horseradish into 2 or 3 tablespoons of buttermilk and let it infuse for 2 or 3 hours, then strain and apply.

Upper lip wrinkles and upper lip lines can be helped with a Papaya "milk" exfoliation (see Papaya in the descriptions), followed by an application of vitamin E as a moisturizer.

Cold sores are soothed with an astringent mixture of Alum root water that has had tincture of Camphor added to it. (See also Chapter XIV.)

Lips are tender and delicate, and mixtures of vitamins C, E, lanolin, and Camphor work well on them if they are dry or chapped.

CHAPPED LIPS

Melt 2 t. beeswax with 4 t. of Apricot oil and ½ t. of Camphor. Stir until the Camphor is dissolved and pour into a small jar. Use whenever necessary. Most chapped lips recipes are just variations on this same theme.

CHAPPED LIPS #2

Beeswax 4 oz., Camphor 2 T., melted together with 5 oz. Olive oil and 1 T. glycerin. Beat until cold.

CHAPPED LIPS #3, More Complicated

Macerate together with the back of a wooden spoon in a small nonmetal pan ¼ oz. each of gum Benzoin, Storax, a chopped red Apple, a small bunch of black Grapes, 4 oz. sweet butter. Add 2½ oz. beeswax and simmer until the wax is melted, and everything is well mixed. Strain out the solids and discard them and beat the remainder until cool. Grease a muffin tin and spoon the mixture into the tin. Then store away for future use.

Your *mouth* and *teeth* also need loving care and attention. Terrible bad breath that mouthwash and toothbrushing do not cure is no doubt the result of an inadequate diet and bad dental hygiene. Try going to a dentist and adding lots of Parsley to your diet as well as using a chlorophyll mouthwash. *Mouthwash* that will tighten loose gums and refresh the breath can easily be made. In ½ cup 100-proof vodka, add 1 oz. of powdered Myrrh. Shake together daily for 10 days, strain through cheesecloth, add oil of Clove to smell. When needed dilute some of the tincture with water and rinse out your mouth. I wouldn't drink too much, however, though this can be used as often as necessary as a mouthwash.

My French relatives say that the first swig of wine should always be swooshed around the mouth as a cleansing astringent mouthwash and then spat out. Then the next swig will really taste as it should.

Infusion of Peppermint or Lavender is refreshing as a mouthwash; salt and soda scented with Mint, Birch, or Clove oil is a cheap and effective toothpowder, rather abrasive for some. Mix salt and soda with mucilage of Quince seed plus Myrrh powder to use as toothpaste. Or add Orris powder to mucilage of Tragacanth and an essential oil for a different sort of toothpaste. For a breath refreshener, chew Clove buds, Parsley or Cinnamon.

For mouthwash infuse herbs in white wine; herbs such as Spearmint, Licorice, Peppermint, Clove, or Myrrh are especially nice.

Cuttlefish bone, powdered, or pumice stone, powdered, is added to toothpowders as an abrasive; only a very little is needed.

CINNAMON TOOTHPOWDER

½ oz. cuttlefish bone	2 t. Peruvian bark-PO
½ oz. chalk	2 t. Orris root-PO

Mix all together and sift through a fine sieve. This may be colored with Beet juice and scented with a few drops oil of Cinnamon.

A RECEIPT TO CLEAN THE TEETH AND GUMS, AND MAKE THE FLESH GROW CLOSE TO THE ROOT OF THE ENAMEL

Take an ounce of Myrrh in fine powder, two spoonfuls of the best white Honey, and a little green Sage in fine powder; mix them well together, and rub the teeth and gums with a little of this Balsam every night and morning.

—The Toilet of Flora, 1779

DITTO, TO STRENGTHEN THE GUMS AND FASTEN LOOSE TEETH

Dissolve an ounce of Myrrh as much as possible in half a pint of Red Wine and the same quantity of Oil of Almonds: Wash the mouth with this fluid every morning. This is also an excellent remedy against worms in the teeth.

—The Toilet of Flora, 1779

AN APPROVED RECEIPT AGAINST THAT TROUBLESOME COMPLAINT, CALLED THE TEETH SET ON EDGE

Purslain, Sorrel, Sweet or Bitter Almonds, Walnuts, or burnt Bread, chewed, will certainly remove this disagreeable sensation.

—The Toilet of Flora, 1779

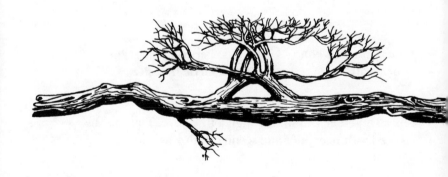

TOOTHBRUSHES CAN BE MADE

By cutting Licorice or Lucern or Marshmallow roots into pieces six inches long, and then boiling them in water for a long time; these are then drained, the ends carefully slit with a pen knife and the brushes dried. Dip your brush into some tooth powder and brush your teeth.

Throats can be considerably improved in their appearance if a pencil is rolled back and forth between the teeth several times a day. Sit up straight, head up and shoulders back when you perform this simple exercise.

The throat area can be exceedingly smoothed with frequent applications of vitamin E. Try massaging a fresh Avocado pit in circles on your throat. Make a cream of 1 T. Avocado or ripe Banana mashed with a teeny bit of anhydrous lanolin and apply generously to the throat area. Massé the cream in with the pit.

Artichokes also contain nourishing materials for the

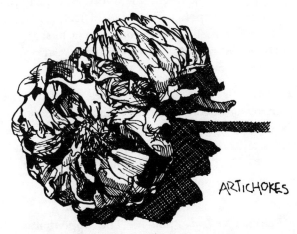

ARTICHOKES

"it mighta choked artie but it aint gonna choke me" - little rascals, 1930's skin. Cook your chokes in water, Celery tops, and Parsley plus 1 T. Olive oil per choke. Eat the Artichokes and save one heart for your throat. Mash ¼ of the heart with 1 t. organic whole egg mayonnaise. Use this beneficial cream to gently massage into the throat area with upward and outward movements. Leave it on for 10 minutes and give yourself a facial sauna so that the Artichoke cream can penetrate, or wipe off the excess and leave the residue on overnight. Then rinse your face and throat and spray with mineral water.

Behind-the-ear blackheads can be removed with a hot compress of Parsley juice placed over the area until the skin is soft and the pores are open.

Or make a solution of 1 tablespoon epsom salts, 1 drop white iodine, and ½ cup of boiling Violet water. Keep the solution hot, dip cotton balls into it and place them on the blackhead; press the blackhead out by spreading the fingers on either side. Don't ever press directly down on a blemish for you might spread the infection; instead press from the sides and up. Because it is so difficult to get to this area of the body ask help from your wife or husband (boy or girl friend will also do). After removing, astringe with Lemon juice or buttermilk.

Natural cosmetics The juice that issues from the Birch-Tree, when wounded with an augur in spring, is detersive and excellent to clear the complexion: the same virtue is attributed to its distilled water. Some people recommend Strawberry-water; others the decoction of Orpiment,[1] and some Frog-spawn water.

—*The Toilet of Flora,* 1779

Or, as *Delightes for Ladies* puts it: "The sappe that issueth out of a Birch tree in great abundance, being opened, in

---

[1]Orpiment is a mineral containing arsenic or the flowers of *Sedum acre.*

March or Aprill, with a receiver of glasse set under the boring thereof to receive the same, doth perform the same most excellently, & maketh the skin very cleer. This sap will dissolve pearle; a secret not known unto many."

Proper breathing is essential for health and handsomeness. It takes just 10 concentrated minutes a day. You could be giving yourself a facial at the same time: Lie down with your legs raised. Breathe in through the nostrils and let the air expand into your abdomen rather than into your lungs, breathe in 7 seconds, hold it for 3 and exhale slowly through the mouth.

For a quick face massage while showering, let a warm water spray flow over your face for 5 minutes. This is very stimulating. You can follow your Shower Facial Massage with an astringe of ice. First cover your skin with flannel or muslin and rub the ice over the fabric and *not* directly over your skin. If you rubbed your skin directly with ice it could cause enlarged blood vessels.

Face fresheners of sparkling mineral water are also nice. Try Évian, Vichy, or Perrier. Fill a plant mister with the water and spray the face after applying make-up to set it, after washing to freshen it and after swimming to remove salt.

Placenta has a reputation in cosmetics as an incomparable moisturizer and wrinkle reducer and is used effectively in medicine. When I had my baby I was urged by some of my more adventurous friends to make use of this wonderful opportunity to experiment with the placenta as a cosmetic. But I managed to resist the temptation to use it, and frankly I think fresh herbs on the face are infinitely more aesthetic and pleasing than fresh placenta.

For a fresh complexion leave your windows open at night even when it is really cold or sleep on a screened sleeping porch, and keep the air moist in your house to keep your skin moist.

UNCLE ED'S SECRET OF HEALTH AND BEAUTY

I went to visit Uncle Ed when I was young and instructive but he was so old that before I could show him where it was at, he forgot what he was looking for. But he died only when he was very old, and his secret for youthful vigor was to walk outside in the snow naked every night and after shaving, wipe his face with icewater or snow, or take a cold shower daily. He told me this in the Laurentian Mountains in January of 1960 when the temperature dropped to minus 40° at night and never went above 0° in the day. Needless to say, he practiced what he preached.

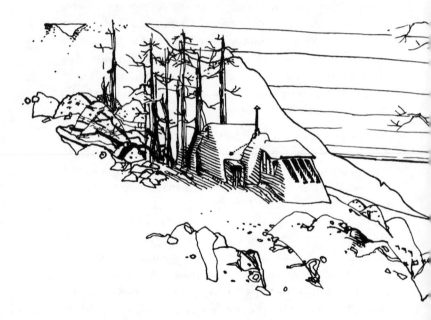

Chapter XIII

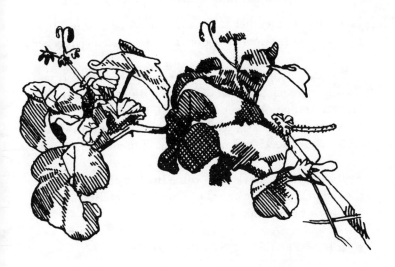

Make-up and Lipsticks

IF YOU EAT well, sleep well, and exercise well you will find
that there is no need to use cosmetics that cover and coat
your skin with artificial colors and textures; your complexion will be so healthy and glowing that it will have its own
color. There are a few botanicals that are useful as face or
lip glosses to give the skin that outdoor sunny look even
when it is in a cold wintry office. And the nice thing about
these cosmetics is that they blend with one's own skin color.
So try them and see and adjust the ingredients to suit
yourself. Less herb for less color, more herb for more
color.

BASIC MAKE-UP RECIPE

> 1 oz. dye herb infused in 4 oz. oil for 2 weeks.
> Heat gently until desired color is reached.
> Strain.
> ¼ oz. yellow beeswax or Cocoa butter

Melt the two together in a small nonmetal pot and beat until cold with a wooden spoon. Put up in a small jar, cover and store away for use.

You can obtain various hues by using the intensely colored herbs such as Parsley, Black or Blue Malva flowers, Henna, Indigo, Alkanet, Cochineal, Red Saunders, Gallnuts, Sassafras bark, Golden Seal, Goldenrod, Black Alder, Sage, Beets, Jamaica flowers, Cinnamon, or Cloves.

Eyebrows can be darkened with a thick decoction of Sage cooked in an iron pot or a Gall-nut decoction. Rub into the eyebrows as often as necessary.

The old herbals also have many eyebrow recipes, one such from *The Toilet of Flora* is as follows:

TO CHANGE THE EYEBROWS BLACK

Rub them frequently with ripe Elder-berries. Some use burnt Cork, or Cloves burnt in the candle; others prefer the Black of Frankincense, Rosin, and Mastic. This Black will not melt nor come off by sweating.

Plain ordinary tea is a useful ingredient in cosmetics not only as an astringent but also to give the skin a sunny look. Make black tea double strength using tea bags. Rub the drained tea bag over a clean face every morning and eventually your skin color will assume an orangy glow.

For darker skin take fresh Carrot juice, apply to your face with cotton balls. This will give your skin an orangy suntanned look. Carrot juice might not be acceptable for fair complexions, however.

Artificial light has a yellowing effect on the skin but pink tends to warm up color. So in the evening:

TO COLOR CHEEKS CARNATION PINK

Mix ½ qt. of white wine together with 1½ oz. gelatin dissolved in a bit of hot water or 2 oz. glycerin, add 1 oz. bruised Nutmeg, 3 oz. honey, and some red Saunders and Alkanet. Shake together daily and when the color is right, strain and pat on the cheeks whenever necessary.

LIPSTICK IN A POT

Soak 2 T. Alkanet root in 4 oz. of Sesame or wheat germ oil for 2 weeks (or less for less color). Melt 4 T. Cocoa butter or yellow beeswax in a small pot slowly and add the strained and drained oil. Beat together until cold and put up in a small jar.

ASTRINGENT FACE GLOSS AFTERSHAVE

1. In ¼ cup Witch Hazel, add ¼ oz. Jamaica flowers.
2. In ¼ cup hot water, add ¼ cup Henna for brown color, or Alkanet for rosy color.
3. After a few hours drain and strain both mixtures. Save the liquid.
4. Make Quince gel of the Henna water by adding 1 T. Quince.
5. Now take the ¼ cup Witch Hazel from step 1, add 1 t. glycerin, 1 T. Henna Quince gel.
6. Mix all together and add scent if you like, such as Peppermint, 1 drop, or Lemon, a few drops.
7. Pat on the face as a healing, coloring lotion.

LIP GLOSS FOR SKIERS

Melt together 1 oz. beeswax and 3 oz. Almond or Apricot oil, add 1 t. Alkanet and some Camphor. Beat until cold.

LIP OR CHEEK GLOSS

Add 1 t. or more Alkanet root or Henna or Red Saunders to Almond oil and infuse for 10 days. Strain. Melt together 1 oz. beeswax and 4 oz. Alkanet-colored Almond oil, and beat until cold.

DARK RUBY RED LIPS OR ROUGE

Infuse Jamaica flowers in Rosewater until it is dark red. Heat some powdered Alkanet in coconut oil until dark red. Strain the Rosewater and the oil, mix, add a bit of melted Cocoa butter and beat together until cold. For darker color yet, add Black Malva flowers to the Alkanet and soak for several days before straining.

PICK UP PINK FOR GLOWING CHEEKS

Juice a small Beet, remove all the large particles, and mix together 1 t. Beet juice and 1 t. glycerin. Pat on the face for a nice glowing color.

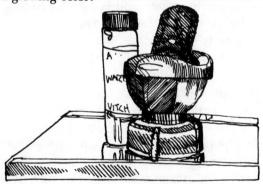

GREEN EYE SHADOW

Heat Parsley in oil. Say 1 oz. Parsley to 4 oz. oil. Heat gently until the oil is dark green. Strain out the Parsley. Add 1 oz. or less of yellow beeswax to the oil, and some chlorophyll for darker color. Heat only until the beeswax is melted and then beat until well incorporated and cold. Put up in a small pot.

GRAPE COLORED EYE SHADOW

Use the above recipe but substitute Black Malva flowers and Alkanet for the Parsley.

SIMPLE AFTERSHAVE FOR A GLOSSY COLOR

Simply infuse Jamaica flowers directly into Rosewater in a ratio of 1:1. Strain and pat on the cheeks. This is also great for ladies as a mild freshener.

GLOSSY BROWN COLORS

Mix a tablespoon of Green Eye Shadow with a like quantity of Pink Lip Gloss.

FACE POWDERS OF DIFFERENT COLORS

Mix any of the following powdered herbs in proportions and combinations to suit your needs: Parsley, Camomile, Corn silk, Orris root, Orange peel, Lemon peel, Jamaica flowers, Lavender, Blue Malva, or Licorice root.

EGGSHELL POWDER FOR FACE OR BODY

Gather together several dozen white eggshells cleaned and dried. Place them in a strong paper bag or wrap in butcher paper and roll them with a rolling pin until crushed and powdery. Sift through a fine lawn sieve several times or grind to a powder in a seed grinder and then sift. Use only the finest powder that goes through the sieve.

You can create colored powders by sifting in various proportions of brown eggs or by sprinkling the eggshell powder with Jamaica flower-colored-Rosewater. Beet

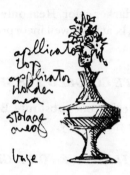

juice, or Carrot juice and then shaking the powder completely and resifting.

You can scent the eggshell powder by sprinkling a few drops of any essence you like on it, shaking the powder in a jar and letting it sit and the scent develop for 2 weeks before using.

Chapter XIV

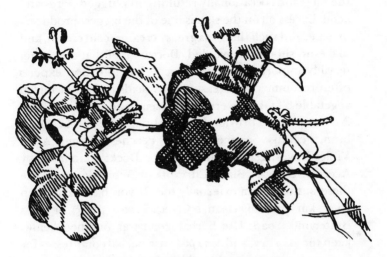

Special Problems:

Acne, Cold Sores, Herpes, Psoriasis, The Pox, Freckles, Pimples, Pustules, Pores, Wrinkles, and Face Peeling

ACNE

GOOD NUTRITION and plenty of regular rest and exercise will go a long way to alleviate a good many of the above problems. But even the most dedicated "Healthy" will occasionally have facial breakouts. It is very difficult to keep a handsome complexion in the midst of the dirty air and soot that abounds in our cities and even in our countrysides today. Acne usually begins in adolescence as a

233

result of increased hormone production which stimulates the oil glands occasionally resulting in plugged pores and acne. Excess oil on the skin is one of the biggest producers of acne, and such things as greasy creams, cold cream, and make-up should be avoided. Doctors feel that diet is not terribly important in curing acne but nutrition experts often recommend increasing fatty acids (1-2 T. of mixed vegetable oil taken every day), niacin, and vitamins C and A. Niacin can be provided by Rice bran, Rice polish, Wheat bran, Peanuts, Sesame Seed, or Peaches; vitamin A, by Violet leaves, Dandelion leaves, or Dock; vitamin C, by Acerola, Guavas, Black Currants or Violet leaves. Take these but use them externally too. If you have acne keep your skin sparkling clean, try Neca 7 soap (pH 7), or Swiss Buttermilk Soap. Use herbal steams as outlined below, keep the skin dry, and *don't pick;* use herbal compresses for the stubborn spots and blackheads, and use herbal masks in the tub.

ACNE HERBAL STEAM

Make a mixture of the herbs listed below in equal proportions and use them according to the steam directions in Chapter VII. You will need about 2–4 T. of herbs per steam. Steam as often as necessary.

Licorice root	Dandelion
Violet leaves, fresh if possible	Dock
Comfrey root	White Willow bark

ACNE HERBAL STEAM #2

Mix equal quantities of the following herbs and use 2–4 T. Steam.

Fennel seed Comfrey leaf
Black currant leaves Dandelion

You can also use the liquid throughout the day as a compress.

ACNE FACIAL MASK

Mash a Guava, strain out the juice, use the pulp on your clean skin while taking a sunbath or sitting in the tub, rinse it off after 10–20 minutes with warm water, then rinse with the Guava juice and then with cool water. You can substitute Black Currants or Violets for the Guava. The pulp of these mashed fruits and herbs loosen the blackheads and help to dry up the pimples.

ACNE COMPRESS

Cook a chopped-up white Onion in a little water and apply the hot pulp several times throughout the day to the pimples. To make a compress, macerate the botanical in a bit of water and bring to a boil. Dip a soft cloth into the water and sponge over the face. Besides Onions, which contain sulfur, you can also use boric acid crystals, Birch bark, Wintergreen, Dandelion, Parsley, Comfrey, Kale, or Watercress.

FRUIT AND HONEY ACNE MASK

Put some honey in the palm of your hand (Sage or Clover honey is preferable), and add enough powdered or mashed cooked Peaches to make a paste. While showering or bathing apply this honey paste to your clean warmed or steamed dry face and pat it all over, especially on the bumps. Take your shower or bath and finally wash it off.

ANOTHER ACNE COMPRESS

Use these herbs every morning for 10 minutes as a compress. Equal parts of Burdock, Marshmallow root, Blue Malva, fresh Onion, and Sage. Mix together.

Remember that "Perseverance furthers." There are no overnight magical cures for acne nor for any other cosmetic problem. Use a combination of the above remedies for some months before you decide that they don't work. Be persistent.

FOR A BAD BUMPY SKIN IN GENERAL

Herbal steams, facial waters, and compresses of the following herbs are most efficacious: Narcissus root water, Burdock tea both internally and externally, Broomrape lotion, Basil tea both internally and externally, and Dandelion and Elder flower tea as a beverage taken several times daily.

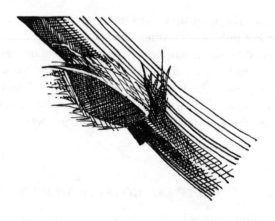

PATCH SOUP NATIONAL ABANDONED

FRECKLES

Freckles can be gradually but not completely erased by external application of the following herbal washes: fumitory water, Solomon seal water, Strawberry leaf water, fumitory water mixed with liquid vitamin C, Lemon juice and honey, boiled Ivy leaves in wine, freshly grated Horseradish infused in yogurt and the yogurt applied daily until the desired results are achieved, and the following old-fashioned formulas:

TO HELP A FACE THAT IS RED OR PIMPLED

Dissolve common Salt in the juice of Lemons, and with a linen cloth pat the patient's face that is full of heat or pimples. It cureth in a few dressings. Or,

TO TAKE AWAY THE FRECKLES IN THE FACE

Wash your face, in the wane of the Moone with a sponge, morning and evening, with the distilled water of Elder-leaves, letting the same dry into the skin. Your water must be distilled in May. This from a Traveller, who hath cured himself thereby.

—*Delightes For Ladies*

Or, from *The Toilet of Flora*, another old marvelous receipt book, we have the following:

TO REMOVE FRECKLES

Take Houseleek and Celandine, of each an equal quantity; distil in a sand heat, and wash with the distilled water.

WRINKLES

Wrinkles on the face can best be helped by diet, adding several tablespoons of brewer's yeast to the food every day, external applications of vitamin E[1] to the wrinkles, Elder flower wash, and this wonderful secret from *The Toilet of Flora*:

A SECRET TO TAKE AWAY WRINKLES

Heat an Iron Shovel red hot, throw on it some Powder of Myrrh, and receive the smoke on your face, covering the head with a napkin to prevent its being dissipated. Repeat this operation three times, then heat the Shovel again, and when fiery hot pour on it a mouthful of White Wine. Receive the vapour of the Wine also on your face, and repeat it three times. Continue this method every night and morning as long as you find occasion.

SPECIAL WRINKLE CREAM

   2 oz. White Lily root juice
   1 oz. beeswax
   2 oz. Orange flower honey

Melt this all together in a small pan, beat until cold. Apply every night and leave on until the next morning.

WRINKLE REMOVER

It is asserted also that the distilled water of green Pineapples takes away wrinkles, and gives the complexion an air of youth.

TO ERASE MARKS OF THE MOTHER, ON ANY PART OF THE BODY

Steep in vinegar of Roses, or strong white wine vinegar, Borage roots stripped of their small adhering fibers, and let them stand to infuse 12 or 14 hours. Bathe the part

---

[1]Here again, dermatologists do not agree with this but it is my personal experience that vitamin E causes wrinkles to become less prominent.

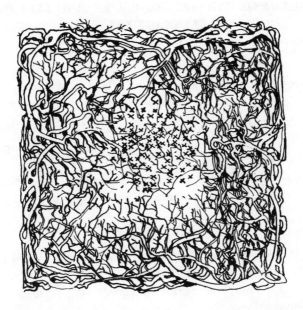

affected frequently with this infusion, and in time, the marks will totally disappear.

Blackheads can be removed by all the previously mentioned blackhead remedies including herbal steams, and also by applying compresses of Lupin seeds mashed up with Lemons, Solomon seal water, Artichoke leaves as an internal and external tea, Apricots mashed in honey and applied as a mask, fresh Tansy leaves soaked in buttermilk and then buttermilk applied as often throughout the day as needed.

Beauty grains of Almond meal, Oatmeal, or Cornmeal moistened with buttermilk or yogurt and used several times a week as a scrub are terrific. Cornmeal mixed with Corn juice is especially cleansing. Whiteheads, called milia, and blackheads are the same except that the whitehead has opened and the air has oxidized the oil, causing a blackhead. If the oil empties under the skin it causes a large reddish area.

BLACKHEAD, WHITEHEAD, PIMPLE, AND BLEMISH BEVERAGE TEA

½ oz. Red Clover
½ oz. Dandelion leaf
½ oz. Comfrey leaf

½ oz. Burdock root
½ oz. Sassafras root
1 oz. Violet leaves and flower

Mix all together and make a strong tea of 1 T. per 1 cup of boiling water. Drink this tea throughout the day and apply the excess as a compress.

Decoctions of Patience, Pimpernel, Fennel, Horsebeans, or Licorice are also used as a daily wash.

MILIA REMOVER

Fill a muslin bag with salt and scrub the milia with it or scrub with the bag and a fine natural bristle complexion brush. The complexion brush and green soap is also useful to remove the milia.

PIMPLE LOTION

Mix together 4 oz. Orange flower water with 1 oz. tincture of Benzoin in a bottle. Because the tincture is made of alcohol this is very drying and should be applied with restraint throughout the day. Shake the bottle each time you wish to use the lotion.

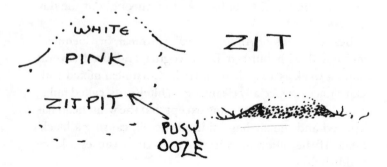

Pores can be refined by other means also; a mushy mask of brewer's yeast with a dab of mayonnaise on a clean face is very stimulating to the circulation. First steam clean your face with herbs, apply the mask, and then wash off with warm water and astringe with Elder flower water or Yarrow water. Brewer's yeast is very stimulating and often cannot be used by really delicate skins. Stimulation can be reduced by oils such as mayonnaise, and increased by such things as Mint, yogurt, or water.

Yarrow water is a potent astringent in cosmetics, and hot compresses are very effectual in aiding the eradication of the dread blackhead. Meals such as Cornmeal mixed with water or yogurt, Almond meal for bleaching plus Lemon juice for additional bleaching, and Barley meal pack are all used to refine and texturize the pores. Herb waters made from Parsley, Marshmallow root, Comfrey, or Fennel seed, or combinations are also exceedingly good for clogged pores. To make these waters for immediate use drop a handful of the herb in boiling water and *simmer* for a few minutes. Let the herbs infuse until cool enough to use. Apply the liquid with cotton balls for 10–15 minutes as often throughout the day as you like. Make the infusion fresh every day or so.

Herpes simplex, also called herpes, cold sores or fever blisters. The trigger situation for a herpes attack can be decreased resistance, poor nutrition, too much sun, or psychic stress. Herpes is caused by the virus *Herpesvirus hominis* and can be cured by better nutrition, keeping the lesion dry, applying cold dressings, and avoiding prolonged soaking (such as in the bath). Herbal relief can be obtained from dabbing on tincture of camphor at the first sign of the sore.

HERPES COMPRESS OR LOTION

1 oz. Borage flowers, fresh if possible	1 oz. Celandine
	1 oz. Marshmallow root
1 oz. White Willow bark	1 oz. Comfrey root

Mix the above herbs together. When you wish to make a lotion, take 1 small handful of the mixed herbs and put in a pot. Add 1 small sliced and mashed yellow Apple and pour over the whole 2 cups of boiling water. Let it infuse until cool, then bring to boil and simmer for 5 minutes. Let cool, then strain through cheesecloth. Use the cold, mashed, strained mixture as a compress on the herpes for 10 minutes night and morning and dab on the cold or ice-cold liquid throughout the day. This should last 1–3 days in the refrigerator.

A SIMPLE HERPES COMPRESS

Can be made by applying a slice of fresh yellow Apple to the inflamed area whenever necessary.

Dermatitis Urbis is a phrase coined by Dr. Irwin Lubowe, Clinical Professor of Dermatology at New York Medical College. It describes a condition of the skin due to continual exposure to air pollution. Here, again, the cure is better nutrition, absolute cleanliness of the skin, and healing herbal lotions. You can use many of the lotion and herbal facial steaming recipes already described but here are two more:

HERBAL SAUNA FOR CITY DIRTY SKIN

Wash your face with neutral soap, leave it damp and steam clean the skin as often as it feels good with the following mixture: 1 oz. each of Camomile, Licorice, Fennel, Parsley, Comfrey root, Comfrey leaf, Peppermint, and Thyme.

Use a small handful each time you steam and afterwards
rinse with warm water and astringe with herbal water or
Rosewater. Stay indoors for at least an hour before going
out.

Dr. Lubowe has formulated a protective cream but you
can make one yourself from the following recipe:

CITY SKIN LOTION

1–3 oz. anhydrous lanolin
1 dab of beeswax
3 oz. of the liquid from the
  above facial sauna,
  strained

1 t. liquid chlorophyll (or
  less)
1 oz. liquid vitamin C
several drops of Lemon oil

Melt the lanolin and the wax together, take off the heat
and add the herbal water, beat together, add chlorophyll,
the vitamin C, and several drops of Lemon oil and beat
continually until thoroughly incorporated and cold.
Spoon into a small jar for use. If the texture doesn't suit
you, remelt and add some oil, about 1 oz., and then beat
until cold. You could also add the contents from several
capsules of vitamins A and E.

CITY SKIN LOTION #2

Macerate and soak in 4 oz. Rosewater for 24 hours ½ oz.
Parsley and ½ oz. Peppermint. Strain and to the liquid add
2 oz. melted anhydrous lanolin and 1 oz. liquid vitamin C.
Beat until thoroughly incorporated, add a few drops of
Lemon oil, and beat until cold.

The word *eczema* refers to a number of different types of
itchy skin diseases which can occur on the face, elbow or
knee creases, wrists or back of the hands (for some this
latter is called "dishpan" hands). The tendency to eczema
is inherited and usually occurs in families that have a

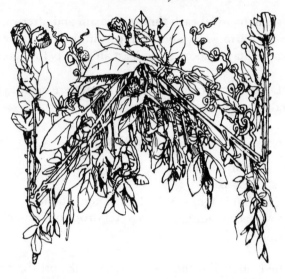

history of allergic problems such as hay fever or asthma. The condition can be aggravated by wool, extremes in temperature, or tension. Persons with eczema tend to have dry skin, and so dry weather, too many showers or baths, and strong or acid soaps, which further dry out the skin, tend to make the eczema worse. Besides the treatments that a dermatologist will prescribe for eczema, there are many herbs that can be effective. You must moisturize the skin to keep it soft, restrict soap bathing, or bathe in herbs using Oatmeal as a scrub instead of soap. Commercial preparations, designed to be used for cleansing those who have eczema, such as Acnaveen, contain such things as sulfur, salicylic acid, and hexachlorophene. You can approximate such a bar using herbs as follows:

ECZEMA HAND AND BODY CLEANSING PASTE

Make a strong decoction of Kale or Watercress, Orange peel, Comfrey root, and White Willow bark using 1 oz. of the mixed herbs to 1 cup of water. Strain the water and add ½ cup finely powdered Oatmeal. Make a mucilage of

Quince or Tragacanth and add enough of the Oatmeal-herb water to make a paste. You can then apply this paste as a compress or use it as a cleansing solution when you take a bath. The Kale and Watercress contain large amounts of sulfur, the Oatmeal is soothing, the Comfrey contains the healing substance allantoin, the White Willow bark contains salicylic acid, and the Orange peel is both aromatic and antiseptic.

ECZEMA BATH OIL

1 oz. crushed Comfrey root
2 oz. Kale, Watercress, Brussels Sprouts, or 1 fresh Onion

1 oz. White Willow bark
1 oz. Echinacea or Gold- en Seal
½ cup white wine

Place the herbs in a 2-quart pot and pour over it ½ cup white wine. Macerate with a wooden spoon and infuse for an hour or so. Add 1 quart of mixed vegetable oil and bring to a boil. Simmer until all the wine cooks off. Stir and smell it constantly. When the wine cooks off in about 20–30 minutes, turn off the heat and let it infuse until cold. Strain through a sieve, then cheesecloth. Squeeze the cheesecloth to get out all of the oil. Let it settle until the oil is clear or almost clear and has a sediment at the bottom. Decant the oil, add up to a cup of wheat germ oil. You can add Wintergreen oil to scent it or crystals of menthol. Use this oil to moisturize your skin or as a bath oil.

ECZEMA BATH

Use a neutral soap such as Neutrogena or Neca 7 or make a tar soap as outlined in Chapter XI. Avoid bathing as much as possible but when you do bathe, add plants such as Comfrey root, White Willow bark, Wintergreen, Bay leaf, Onions, Cabbage, Cranberry, Marshmallow root, and col- loidal or plain Oatmeal in a bag. Scrub with the Oatmeal bag (make the bag of cheesecloth or muslin and add cooked Oatmeal).

Nutritionists feel that diet is very important in dealing with eczema and would add such things as biotin, yeast, PABA, inositol, B6, and fats. Inositol can be obtained in Grapefruits, Oranges, wheat germ, and nuts; B6 in Rice polish, wheat germ, Cabbage; PABA in Rice polish, Rice grain, or wheat germ.

ECZEMA APPLICATION

Apply the gel from a section of the Aloe leaf to soothe and heal whenever you like throughout the day.

ECZEMA COMPRESS

Morning and evening use a 10-minute compress of the following herbs: California Poppy, Brier Rose petals and leaves, Linden, Nettle, Comfrey root, Fuchsia flowers.

ECZEMA LOTION

Grate raw fresh Horseradish into yogurt, buttermilk, or sour milk. Let it infuse for some hours before using. Refrigerate. Dab on whenever the itch gets intolerable. After a day or so, when the milk or yogurt has acquired the properties of the Horseradish, strain out the Horseradish and keep the milk for use. This preparation sometimes burns slightly when applied; in such a case, rinse off with cool water for a few minutes and pat the area dry.

Psoriasis is a skin disease (it tends to be inherited) in which the epidermis makes skin at about 10 times the normal rate. The skin, instead of becoming flat and smooth, bunches up into scales. It usually affects elbows, knees, or the scalp, palms, or soles of the feet. Dermatologists feel that no dietary factors are involved but nutritionists feel that the addition of fatty acids and zinc and the exclusion of food preservatives and additives are helpful. The treatment is to keep the skin soft with preparations containing tar, salicylic acid, allantoin (Comfrey), lanolin, tar shampoos, and soaps, and medicated baths containing oils and tar. Also direct application of *Aloe vera*.

PSORIASIS SALVE

1 oz. White Willow bark or Wintergreen	1 oz. Orange peel
1 oz. Comfrey root	1 oz. Echinacea

Make a strong decoction of the above herbs, simmering for at least 20 minutes. Cool and strain. Use the herbs as a compress and to 2–4 parts of the liquid add 1 part of melted anhydrous lanolin. Beat together until cold. The rest of the liquid and herbs can be dumped into your bath to medicate it. This salve is very potent, not pungent, thick and muddy-colored, but highly effective. I make it in a small enamel gravy pot that holds about 8 fluid ounces. If it seems too thick for easy application soften a bit in a heated metal spoon to facilitate penetration.

PSORIASIS BATH HERBS

Herbs such as Marshmallow root, Comfrey root, Pansy, Birch bark, White Willow, Wintergreen, Clovers, Camomile, or Seaweed are useful additions to the bath, especially combinations that provide a healing agent such as Comfrey root with a salicylic acid herb such as White Willow bark. You can use a tar soap such as that outlined in Chapter XI.

PSORIASIS SHAMPOO

Make the shampoo with the herbs as listed above and according to directions outlined in Chapter XV.

Facial peeling, also called exfoliation, is easily accomplished at home. It simply means to remove the outer layer of the skin, thereby removing surface blemishes and leaving your skin pink and shiny.

LOOFAH SCRUB

The easiest method is to wash your face, leave it damp, and scrub it in circular motions with a small loofah or hemp or horsehair mitt. You can apply a bit of Cornmeal, soap, or Oatmeal to the loofah or mitt.

COMPLEXION BRUSH PEELING

Another method is to steam your skin clean with some medicating herbs such as those listed in Chapter VII and then wash with soap and a complexion brush made of natural bristles. Always rinse with warm water and then with cold to close the pores.

FRUIT PEELERS

Exfoliation using fruits such as Pineapple, Tomato, Lime, or Lemon is accomplished by first steam cleaning the face with diaphoretic herbs (Chapter VII), applying the drained and mashed pulp or juice of the fruit to the skin, and then massaging it in circular motions. Rinse with warm and then cool water and follow with an herbal rinse. Your skin will feel soft and delicate.

HONEY PEELERS

The Honey Pat (Chapter IX) is also an excellent peeler. Just keep patting until you can barely remove your finger from the skin. Rinse in warm water and follow with a mineral water rinse or a Camomile water rinse.

CORNY HONEY PEELER FOR FACE OR BODY

1 T. Cornmeal
1 T. Orange honey

Mix the two together in the palm of your hand and apply to a steamed and cleaned face using circular motions. When the honey is tacky, apply a thin layer of yogurt, take a bath or shower and remove when rinsing—first with warm and then with cool water.

THE MAYONNAISE PEEL

This is my favorite peel, and I use it about once a month. Take 1 teaspoon of wheat germ oil (Avocado, Almond, or any other oil may also be used), and massage on the clean face in circular motions with the heel of the hands, then add about 1 teaspoon of herbed water (I use Peppermint water), and massage this in with circular motions and finally add 1 teaspoon of Lime juice (Lemon or Pineapple juice can also be used). Now rub this facial mayonnaise in circular motions, and you will feel little balls of gluck begin

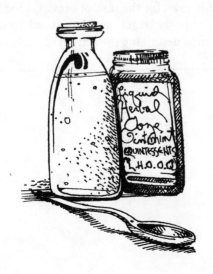

to collect on your hands. Discard the gluck and keep rubbing until your whole face feels smooth. You might want to complete the mayonnaise peel with a quick steam of emollient herbs, a soap and water wash, or an application of Aloe gel.

While writing this Chapter I watched a TV movie about a ghoul with aging skin. Terrific inspiration for psoriasis.

Pores do not really expand and contract; they cannot open and close like windows according to the amount of heat or cold or type of substance that is applied. When we speak of contracting a pore we are using a euphemism for a physiological action that would require many words to describe. When a pore is enlarged it may be made to appear smaller and this we call contraction. What actually happens is that an astringent or substance is applied and an edema forms around the pore. This puffed-up skin makes it appear as if the pore has "contracted." It takes a long time and much diligent effort to make these pores look smaller or "contracted" all the time. Often this is not possible. However, for the sake of brevity, I too have fallen in with the popular jargon and have used "contract" and "expand" when describing the actions of herbs on the skin.

H IS FOR HAIR

A good head of shiny glossy hair can be achieved simply by treating your hair as kindly as you treat the skin of your face. Feed it with nourishing foods, rest it well, and exercise to condition your whole body and improve its circulation. If you massage your scalp with your fingers in the sun once a day, or as often as possible, it will improve the circulation to the scalp and activate growth. There are

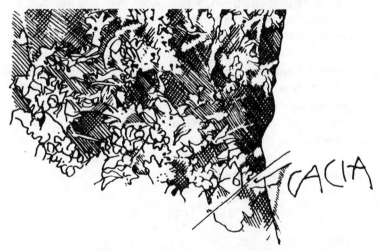

many useful herbs for the hair: Coltsfoot and Fennel to open the pores of the scalp and face; Yarrow, Birch leaves, Speedwell, Comfrey, Horsetail to soothe the scalp and relieve irritations; Camomile, Parsley, Mullein, and Violet to help allergic reactions; Nettle, Arnica, Rosemary, Southernwood, Jaborandi for growth and gloss; Juniper, Pine, Lavender, and Arnica for stimulation and a refreshing fragrance; Horseradish and Wallpepper for strong stimulation; Black Cherry bark, Burdock, Clover, and Rosemary for manageability and gloss; Burdock, Aloe, Cloves for dry or itchy scalp. Check Chapter I under Hair for many more herbs and their hair use.

Bathe your head with seawater and Seaweed to condition the scalp, add eggs to shampoo as a protein conditioner for dry hair, or Lemon juice and cold water as a rinse for oily and unbleached hair. Shampoo regularly but not constantly; brush at least once a day (men too); if you hate brushing then run your fingers through your hair to condition it; condition with Rosemary oil or Lavender oil; keep away from hair dryers, hair sprays, electric curlers; don't go to bed with curlers on and *do* leave a window open; use a natural shampoo, a pure boar bristle brush and a nonplastic comb; if you are female, stay away from hair combs with sharp jagged teeth or those made of plastic; men and women, tie up your hair with anything except rubber bands or plastic covered rubber bands; wear as natural a style as possible, no teasing, back combing or trying to straighten curly hair or curling straight hair; ignore the desire for a permanent, or chemical dyes and other plastic chemical changes to your hair.

Love it and care for it; it will reward you by becoming a glossy healthy frame for your face.

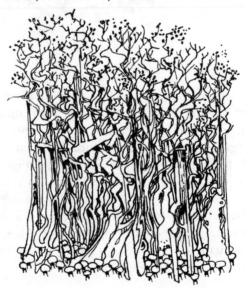

Chapter XV

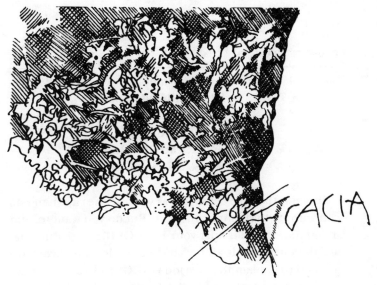

Shampoos

WITH ALL THE TV and magazine commercials about shampoos, what exactly do you *know* about them? What are they made of? Why or how do they work and do they *really* do what the commercials say? Take, for instance, the popular so-called herbal shampoos that make you think of flowers or bathing in streams and how much you'll love the scent. Do they use the synthetic scent to cover up possible nasty aromas that the ingredients might have had before the scent was added? I don't know. Do you? And we all know that herbs are good for the hair: but are herbs, or their synthetic essences, the ingredients in the shampoo?

Northern Petrochemical Company supplies potential customers with suggested formulations for cosmetics and toiletries. One of the most interesting comparisons is that of their suggested formulation of Gel-Type Hair Shampoo and Rug Shampoo. Compare the ingredients:

GEL-TYPE SHAMPOO		RUG SHAMPOO CONCENTRATE
34%	Water	52%
50%	DLS-VARONOL-SLS	40%
8%	CADG-VARION-CADG	4%
	Lauric Isopropanolamide	4%
5%	VARAMIDE-ML1	
3%	20% Salt Solution	

It seems that one could just as well use the rug shampoo concentrate to shampoo the hair. But do you want to, and if you did, would it hurt your hair? Or the rug? But what are these chemicals and what do they do? The brochure goes on to explain that Varion CADG is a foaming agent, emulsifying agent, and is also biodegradable. Varonol is simply described as containing Laury Alcohol Sulfate and a salt; and Varamide, contained only in the hair shampoo, is a thickener and foam stabilizer.

And what about "organic" shampoos with a pH of 4.5–5.5, or neutral? As you know, pH indicates the amount of alkalinity or acidity a substance has. The number 7 indicates neutral, more than 7 is alkaline and less than 7 is acid. Your hair and skin have a slightly acid pH. I know of no soap or soap-like product made by nature that has a pH of 4.5–5.5, the normal pH of the hair. All shampoos with this artificially contrived pH, whether or not they are called "natural" or "organic," are made in laboratories with generally the cheapest possible ingredients.

Let's have a look at these so-called natural shampoos. The usual formula for a commercially made shampoo is roughly this: 44 per cent water; 40 per cent sudsing agent (usually an artificially made substance that makes piles of synthetic suds); 10 per cent foam stabilizer (so that the piles of suds won't engulf you and can be flushed down the drain); 3 per cent emulsifier or stabilizer (to hold all the synthetic ingredients together); 1 per cent protein; 2 per cent preservative (usually formalin and salt); and a touch of artificial perfume to cover up the nasty smell of the preceding chemicals.

In addition, any shampoo smelling of Basil, Roses, or any other heavy-leafed flower or herb is a shampoo scented with a synthetic oil. Now synthetic oils are OK but the cosmetic people should at least tell you when they are using a synthetic instead of a natural perfume. Natural oils from these heavy-leafed botanicals are so expensive that it would be impossible to put enough in the shampoo to get such a strong smell. Avocado oils, too, are expensive, and most "Avocado" shampoos contain just a tiny amount of this—classified as a semidrying oil and thus useful only for oily hair. It would be better to mash an Avocado on your head (which *is* very effective, see pages 263 and 264) than to use a drying Avocado shampoo, and the same can be said for Peppermint shampoo; Peppermint oil is *very drying to the hair,* while the herb, Peppermint, is an emollient and very *soothing*.

A properly made soap has a natural pH close to 7. Olive oil castile has a pH of 7–8. Your hair and skin, if you are healthy, go back to their normal, slightly acid pH in a very short time after you bathe or shampoo with soap. If you are concerned about the pH of your hair or skin, then after you shampoo or bathe you can use a cosmetic vinegar or Rosewater Astringent Lotion (Chapter X) as an acid astringent, or a vinegar or Lemon rinse on the hair. An astringent helps to bring your skin back to its normal, slightly acid pH quickly. There is no need to be sucked in by exaggerated advertising which encourages you to run out and purchase expensive astringents or hair rinses; the finest natural astringents are in your kitchen and include

Lemon juice, Tomato juice, or a vinegar that has had herbs infused in it such as Herbal Vinegar Conditioning Rinse (Chapter XVI).

Herbal Shampoo. Now some shampoos are really made with herbs; botanical plants, green things picked from the earths of the world. These herbs are infused in water and then simmered to extract all their natural good essences; this strained extract is then mixed with a high quality Olive oil castile soap, maybe some protein, and then a touch of natural perfume added. The resultant shampoo is then bottled, the bottles labeled and the labeled bottles delivered to the store; and hopefully, this really natural organic shampoo is fresh, and it will need no emulsifier, sudsing agent, or preservative.

But this type of natural herbal shampoo sometimes solidifies in cold weather or in a cold house. What this means is that without an emulsifier to hold it together, the shampoo will separate into its components, the herbal liquid layer and a solid white soap layer. There is nothing wrong

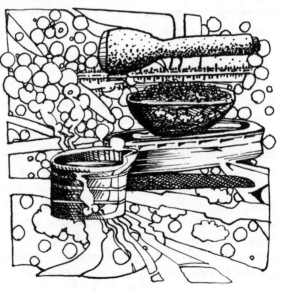

with this or bad about the shampoo; all you have to do is to set the mixture in a warm window, put it into a pot of hot water, or in some other way, gently heat it, and *voilà,* everything will melt, reliquefy, and go back together.

PROPER SHAMPOOING

Too many people use too much shampoo. To avoid this, take about an ounce of your favorite shampoo and mix it with a few ounces of water; mix together well. Use this mixture to shampoo your hair, and it will enable both your hair and the shampoo to last that much longer.

What is the proper procedure for the beauty shampoo? Firstly, wet, WET, your hair thoroughly with warm to hot water; this opens the pores and fills them with water. Then take about half of your water and shampoo mix and pour it slowly over your scalp, and working your hands underneath your wet hair, proceed to massage and scrub your scalp. The hair, itself, hardly needs bothering with as the soap that drips down the hair will take off the extra oil and dirt that is there. The scalp needs most of the cleaning effort. Scrub your scalp with your fingerpads gently and not with your fingernails. If your hair is really dirty, the dirt and oil will depress the sudsing action and you will not have any suds. But scrub your entire scalp diligently and then rinse completely. Rinse again and apply the last half of the soap and water mixture. This time you will probably work up a good head of suds—but suds are not the important thing—your hair might squeak a little and then you know it is clean. Rinse again thoroughly.

It is at this point that I would apply an herb rinse. Some like 1 tablespoon of vinegar to 2 cups of water; blonds like half a Lemon, juiced and added to 2 cups of water. I would prefer an herbal infusion. There are many mixtures that one can use and these recipes follow in Chapters XVI and XVII.

Since I am brown-haired I like to use a mixture of Black Cherry bark for conditioning. Cloves for scent, White Willow bark for scalp problems, and Camomile for highlighting—mix equal parts and then infuse 1 or 2 heaping T. herbs for 5 minutes in 1 cup boiling water; strain, then add an equal amount of cold water and apply to the hair. Keep pouring it on—catching the extra in a pot and repouring until you are bored. Towel dry.

And now, with this clean wet hair, do you immediately attack it with a clean brush and comb. NO, NO, NO, a thousand times NO. NEVER NEVER put a brush or comb to wet hair. Wet hair is just like a stretched out rubber band and trying to comb it will damage and break it. So get out in the sun or walk around your house or apartment to allow it to dry, pull your fingers gently through your hair until it is completely dry. As it dries, its natural elasticity returns and when dry you can then brush or comb to your heart's delight.

Your lovely hair will respond to natural hair care. It takes time and energy but the results are worth the efforts. There are 3 main steps besides a sensible diet, rest, and exercise required in taking care of hair:

1. Shampooing with a natural herbal shampoo.
2. Proper brushing with a natural bristle brush.
3. Correct conditioning.

SHAMPOO RECIPES

GENERAL SHAMPOO RECIPE

To make 8 ounces of shampoo, put 1 ounce or more of mixed herbs in a nonmetal or enamel pot and add 10 ounces or a bit more of spring water—or tap water will do. Bring gently to a boil, lower heat, and gently simmer for 5–10 minutes. Turn off heat and let infuse for 5–10 minutes longer. Strain off the liquid into another pot that contains 1 ounce of good quality Olive oil castile soap,[1] Stir until the soap melts and add 1 or 2 drops of your favorite essential oil. Oil of Clove is nice for dark hair and oil of Lemon or Orange is nice for blonds, but oil of Wintergreen, Birch, Cinnamon, Mint, or anything else that you like will do. Now bottle your genuine herbal shampoo, use sparingly and it will last 1 person from 3–8 weeks.

Where will you find a good quality castile soap? Indiana Botanic carries Conti castile in flakes, and there is also a soap called Hard Water Castile that, when shaved or grated, makes a pretty good castile shampoo.

A good shampoo should contain:

a medicinal or cleansing herb-M
an emollient-E
an herb for color-C
an herb for conditioning-CD
scent-S, if you like

If your hair is oily, you will also need an herb to reduce oiliness; if your hair is dry, an additional emollient herb or herbs that contain one or many of these qualities as follows or in Chapter I.

HAIR GROWTH SHAMPOO

Any of the following herbs are said to stimulate hair growth: Nettle, Maidenhair Fern, Sage, Peach leaf, California Poppy, and Jaborandi. Blonds could use a mixture of California Poppy flowers and Camomile; and brunettes could use any of the plants mentioned while a perfect mixture would be equal quantities of Nettle-CD, Peach leaf-E, Jaborandi-M, and Clove-C+S. Follow the general recipe.

[1]Check Chapter VI for other sources of castile soaplets.

BLOND SHAMPOO FOR LIGHT HAIRS

Any of the following: Camomile, Mullein flower, Calamus, Orange flower, Marigold, Orris root, Quassia chips, Turmeric, or Henna. A good mixture would be equal quantities of Camomile-C+CD, Marigold-E, Quassia chip-M, and maybe Orange peel-S. Follow the general recipe.

BROWN HAIR SHAMPOO

Aloe leaf-M, Maidenhair Fern-M, Yarrow-M, Clove-S, Cassia bark, or any brown plant. A good mixture would be equal quantities of Henna-C, Marigold-E, Camomile-CD, and a touch of Cassia bark-S, and maybe Clove-S. Follow the general recipe.

RED HAIR SHAMPOO

Marigold, Cochineal, Witch Hazel bark, Henna, Clove, Red Hibiscus, Jamaica flowers, or any other red plant. A good mix: Marigold-E+CD, Witch Hazel bark-M+S, and Henna-C. Follow the general recipe.

BRUNETTE SHAMPOO

Rosemary, Cloves, Marjoram, Lavender, Raspberry, Sage, Sassafras, Mint, Comfrey leaf, and also any of the herbs mentioned under brown hair, black hair, or hair growth listed in Chapter I. A good mixture would be Rosemary, Southernwood, Lemon peel, Nettle, and Artichoke leaves. If you want your brunette hair to have a shiny bright light to it, wash it with blond shampoo and rinse it with the herbs mentioned under light hair rinses. Follow the general recipe.

BLUE HAIR SHAMPOO

The herbs Bachelor Button, Blue Malva, and White Camomile flowers are very useful for those lucky persons with hair so white that it looks blue. But they should also realize that their hair is probably very dry, and they should, therefore, add an emollient both in the shampoo and in the conditioning rinse after the shampoo. Both Comfrey root and Blue Malva would be useful emollients so a good mixture for the blue hairs or very white hairs is one made up of equal parts of Comfrey root or Blue Malva, Bachelor Button, and White Camomile. Lavender flowers smell delightful but are best used for people who do not have a dryness problem. Follow the general recipe.

BLACK HAIR SHAMPOO

An excellent mixture would be equal parts of Indigo, Black Malva, and Lavender, with maybe Henna or Cloves added if you wish a reddish highlight. Follow the general recipe.

DRY HAIR SHAMPOO

Any of the following are good: Comfrey root and leaf, Acacia flowers, Red Clover, Melilot, Orange flowers and peel, Elder flowers, and of course, the dietary supplements that are usually prescribed are vitamins A, E, and the fatty acids.

OILY HAIR SHAMPOO

The herbs Orris root, Quassia chips, Lemongrass, Orange leaf, Peppermint, Willow bark, and Witch Hazel bark and leaf. A good mixture would be Quassia chip-M, Lemongrass-CD, Peppermint-S+E, and Willow bark-M in equal proportions. You will probably need to increase your intake of vitamins B_2 and B_6.

DANDRUFF HAIR SHAMPOO

The herbs that are most useful are White Willow bark,

Birch bark, Peppermint, Nettle, Artichoke leaves, Creosote bush, Quassia chips, and Comfrey root or leaf. An excellent combination would be Comfrey leaf-E+CD, Quassia chip-M, Willow or Birch bark-M, and Artichoke or Creosote in equal proportions.

OTHER HERBS EXCELLENT IN SHAMPOO

Acacia flowers, Cowslips, Elder, Kelp, Linden, Juniper berries, Lemon Balm (Melissa), Gentian, Horsetail, Speedwell, and Ginger.

Now you will ask, "But I have brunette hair that has an oily scalp and dry hairs, so what do I do?" Well, actually the answer is easy.[1] Use Chapter I to good advantage. Take one of the dark herbs from the brunette list, like Rosemary or Sage, an emollient like Comfrey root from the dry list, and Willow or Lemongrass from the oily list, then add Red Clover because it is so good for all hair, and make your personal-made-to-order herbal shampoo. If you are blond or light-haired then just make sure that all the herbs you choose from the list are light-colored plants. A good all-around dry hair mixture for light-haired persons is: Quassia chip, Marigold, Camomile, Orange peel, and Lemon peel—all in equal proportions.

Shampoos must clean the hair but not strip it of all its essential oils, and they must take care of your own personal hair problems (see Chapter I); i.e., using egg yolks for fine hair to give it body (just add an egg to your favorite herbal shampoo, or shampoo with the yolk only and rinse com-

---

[1]Obviously, the sebaceous glands are simply out of order and herbs really are just balancers. They act to normalize a condition. There is not really one herb that acts specifically on only one problem. For every problem there are numbers of herbs that can be used. For instance, Lemongrass acts to normalize the sebaceous glands but also seems to be more effective in oily conditions. But since it does normalize it also acts to balance the dry condition and is therefore the perfect herb to use in this example.

pletely with soft water); for dry hair you can add ½ oz. of Almond oil to 1 oz. of your own herbal shampoo, then shampoo, rinse, and rinse again with an herbal vinegar rinse.

DETERGENT SHAMPOO

Hair is unmanageable when a shampoo washes too well. These detergent shampoos remove the dirt as well as the natural oils. Castile shampoos with herbs such as Rosemary, Sage, Thyme, and Camomile are best.

AVOCADO SHAMPOO For Dry or Oily Hair That Needs Body

½ cup herbal castile shampoo (your choice of herbs but you might add Lemon or Lavender for oily hair and Acacia or Clover for dry hair)
½ cup soft water
½ of a mashed Avocado

1. Mix all the ingredients in a blender and shampoo hair in the regular manner; i.e., wet hair completely, apply Avocado shampoo at scalp and to hair, add warm water gradually, working up a lather.
2. Rinse, rinse, rinse with warm water until the hair feels clean and sounds clean (not necessarily squeaky which indicates that *all* the natural oils plus the Avocado oil have been removed).
3. Rinse dry hair with a rinse for dry hair (Chapter XVI, and oily hair with the juice of half a Lemon mixed with water.

Dry shampoos are used and necessary when it is cold or raining or you are in a hurry and want to clean your hair;

try any of the following meals and powders after thoroughly and completely brushing your hair:

1. Rub stone-ground Cornmeal through the hair, one section at a time, rubbing vigorously into the scalp. Brush with a clean brush to get rid of the old hair oils and accumulated dirt and odors.
2. Bean meal, Oatmeal, bran, and Almond meal are also useful as dry shampoos. Often these meals are more easily removed from light rather than dark hair. But with vigorous brushing they can be used by even the darkest haired.
3. Orris root is especially nice on light-colored hair as it both removes the dirt and lightly scents the hair. Try a mixture of Cornmeal and Orris root.
4. Rub your hair section by section with a piece of *clean silk*. This gives body and shine. It is a particularly nice way to dry a child's hair after shampooing. It takes about 30 minutes of vigorous rubbing.
5. Frothy egg whites make an excellent foam to brush through the hair if you don't wish to take the time for a long shampoo—brush the hair, apply the egg-white foam with the fingers, massage the scalp thoroughly, apply all of the foam and let it dry, and then brush it out completely with a clean brush.

NOTES ON HAIR CARE

Shampoo sparingly with an herbal shampoo—never more than 3 times per week. Too much shampooing aggravates oiliness. Cut down shampoo gradually to once a week and also add Lemongrass to the shampoo. Brush oily hair thoroughly once a day as it activates the oil-producing glands and also distributes the oil evenly along the hair shaft to the oil poor ends. For dry split ends singe the ends to seal them. Shampoo dry hair once a week, rinse with an herbal rinse for dry hair and condition daily with Rosemary essential oil for the hair. For healthy hair as well as a healthy body, eat a sensible diet that includes protein and plenty of vitamins and minerals.

As a last word, NEVER NEVER put a brush or comb through your hair while it is wet. Shampoo, rinse, rinse with a conditioning rinse if necessary or with an herbal hair rinse, and then let your hair dry naturally, fluffing it out occasionally with your fingers. When thoroughly dry, condition with Rosemary oil and bend over and brush your hair from nape to ends with a minimum of 100 strokes; good exercise for your hair and your wrists as well.

FIGHT HAIR POLLUTION—Use Herbs for Hair Health.

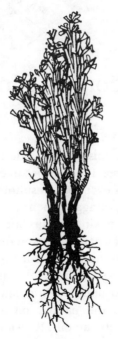

Chapter XVI

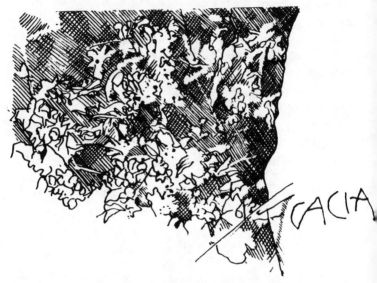

Conditioning Rinses

IF A SHAMPOO washes too well, it can cause the hair to become unmanageable; this usually indicates there is detergent in the shampoo. The hair becomes slick and dries out, but the oil glands overwork, resulting in greasy scalp and the need to shampoo again. Soon you are shampooing every day, not only removing the dirt but also stripping all the natural oils from the hair. Then you find that you need a conditioning rinse to supply the hair with much needed oils that the shampooing removed. Commercial conditioning rinses contain coconut oil and lanolin. Detergent shampooing removes the natural oil and commercial conditioners add nonhuman oils. Ridiculous isn't it? The best shampoos remove only the surface dirt and leave the natural oils; herbal shampoos also give something back to the hair in the form of conditioning agents. These conditioning agents are the *herbs*. Alive, healthy-looking hair needs only a mild cleansing shampoo and an after-shampoo herb conditioning rinse.

The best *conditioners* for hair, whether in the shampoo or in the rinse, are: inner bark of the Wild Cherry tree, Ragwood (also called Ragweed), Nettle, Camomile, Lemongrass, Rosemary, Parsnip root and seeds, and Burdock root.

BASIC CONDITIONING RINSE RECIPE

1. Thoroughly mix your herbs, take about 1–4 heaping T. and drop into a covered nonmetal pot. Add about 1 cup of water.
2. Cover the pot and bring to a boil, lower the heat; *do not boil* but *simmer* for 3–5 minutes.
3. Strain. Add 1 cup cool water to the infusion. Take the strained herbs and put them into your garden or sprinkle onto your potten plants—this makes excellent food and mulch for the plants.
4. Now pour this herbal infusion over your clean wet hair, letting the excess drip into the pot, and pouring and repouring over your head, gently rubbing it into the scalp and letting the liquid drip down the hair shafts. Squeeze out the excess. It is *not* necessary to follow an herbal rinse with a rinse of clear water, but you can do so if you wish. Let your hair air dry or help it along by gently working your fingers through the hair and waving it about in the sun or in the air. When it is completely dry, brush as described in the brushing section.

SUPER BEST CONDITIONER RINSE FOR AFTER SHAMPOO

. . . An Herbal Alternate to the Cream Rinse . . .

Mix 2 oz. Black Cherry bark, 1 oz. Ragweed, and 1 oz. Nettle. These can all be obtained from your local herb store such as Nature's Herb Company in San Francisco on the West Coast, and Kiehl's Pharmacy in New York (for other sources of supply look in Chapter VI). Follow the basic recipe for application.

CONDITIONING RINSE FOR LIGHT HAIR

Mix together equal quantities of Camomile, Marigold, and Acacia flowers if you have them. Follow the basic recipe for application. Store the excess away in a bottle or bag in a cool dark place. Follow the basic rinse recipe.

CONDITIONING RINSE FOR DARK HAIR

Mix together Rosemary, Sage, and Quassia chips in equal quantities. Add a pinch of bruised Cloves. Follow the basic recipe for application and store the excess away in a cool, dark place. Follow the basic rinse recipe.

A GOOD RINSE FOR DANDRUFF

Dandruff conditions can be considerably helped with rinses of any of the following herbs: White Willow bark, Nettle, Birch bark, Artichoke leaves, Creosote bush, and Peyote root. Follow the basic rinse recipe.

ASTRINGENT HAIR RINSE FOR ALL HAIR

Use the rinse to close pores and for dandruff. Mix equal quantities of Witch Hazel bark, White Willow bark, Comfrey root, Licorice root, and either scented Geranium or Rosemary leaf. Take a small handful of the herbs and add ½ qt. of water. Bring to a boil in a small nonmetal pot with a close-fitting lid and *simmer* for up to 20 minutes. Take off the heat until cool enough to use and then strain. Now pour this through your clean, just washed and rinsed hair over and over again, catching what drips off in a basin and repouring through the hair, massaging into the scalp. You may rinse again with cool clear water or leave the herbal rinse on as you wish.

CONDITIONER VINEGAR OR RINSE FOR DARK HAIR AND TO STIMULATE GROWTH

Mix together Rosemary, Nettle, Jaborandi, and Cloves in equal quantities and follow either the basic rinse or vinegar rinse directions.

CONDITIONER RINSE FOR DARK HAIR—TO BRIGHTEN

Mix together Rosemary, Henna, Camomile, and Marigold in equal proportions and apply according to the basic recipe. This is not suitable to the vinegar rinse method.

CONDITIONER RINSE FOR LIGHT HAIR

Mix together Camomile, Orange peel, Marigold flowers, and Yellow Mullein flowers. If the hair is fine and prone to tangles, add the bark of the Black Cherry. Follow the basic conditioning rinse recipe.

HAIR RINSE FOR DRY HAIR

Mix together equal quantities of Acacia, Elder flower, Comfrey root, Clover, and fresh Orange blossoms. Follow the basic rinse recipe.

HAIR RINSE FOR DRY HAIR #2

Mix together equal quantities of Melilot, Cowslip, Comfrey leaf, and Orange peel. Follow the basic rinse recipe.

HAIR RINSE FOR OILY HAIR

Mix together any of the following herbs in equal proportions: Lemongrass, Quassia chip, Artichoke leaves, Lemon
peel and Willow bark. Follow the basic rinse recipe.

OTHER HERBS FOR OILY HAIR

Vinegar rinses containing Pansy, Peppermint, Orris root,
Orange bergamot, Witch hazel, and Birch bark are good
for oily hair as well as for a dry, itchy scalp.

TO CLEAN THE HAIR AND KEEP IT FROM COMING
OUT

> 3 oz. Rosemary leaf
> a lump of baking soda
> 1½ t. Camphor

Put in a pot and cover with 1 qt. of boiling water, cover, and
set aside overnight, strain, add 4 oz. of rum. Apply this to
the roots with cotton balls daily.

CONDITIONER RINSE
OR VINEGAR RINSE TO STIMULATE GROWTH

These herbs have a folk history of stimulating hair growth
when used persistently over a period of time: Peach kernels, Jaborandi, Nettle, Rosemary, and Southernwood.

VINEGAR RINSES

Vinegar rinses are also good for the hair to soften and
condition it and to neutralize the alkalinity of soap. The
same herbs that are used for herbal hair infusions can be
used in vinegar rinses as follows:

1. Mix your herbs together in the quantities you desire.

2. Bring 1 cup of Apple cider vinegar to a boil and pour over 1 oz. of mixed herbs.
3. Cover the container and set aside for a week in a cool, dark place, shaking it daily.
4. Strain out the herbs and store the herbal vinegar.
5. When needed, mix 1 T.–¼ cup of the vinegar (strength depends on how strong a mixture you like) to 1 cup of warm water.
6. Pour the conditioning vinegar through your clean washed hair, catching the excess in a basin, pouring and repouring through your hair.
7. Rinse lightly with cool, clear water.

DAILY CONDITIONERS

The best daily conditioner for your hair is essential oil of Lavender, Basil, or Rosemary. These essential oils and herbs have been used for centuries to condition the hair and promote its growth. Lavender and Basil oils are so expensive, however, that in days past only the richest people or royalty could afford to use them, and so people turned to Rosemary oil which is very effective and has the advantage of being reasonably priced. The smell is quite aromatic and strong at first, but it is very volatile and the initial strong aroma is soon dispersed, leaving only a fresh aromatic smell on your hair. One company packages Rosemary Hair Oil containing about 2 per cent pure oil of Lavender for its richness and to moderate the harsh scent of the Rosemary. But if you will purchase 1 oz. of essential oil of Rosemary and mix it with about ¼ oz. essential oil of Lavender or Basil—whichever scent you prefer—you will get a daily conditioner fit for a king. Rosemary oil conditions the hair, adds luster and gloss without making the hair oily, reduces the amount of snarls and tangles, stimulates growth, and eliminates the need for a cream rinse.

Cream rinses leave the hair limp and weak and coat it with an oily film. Use only a drop or two of the Rosemary or Lavender oil, first on the palm of your hand, then rubbing your palm over your natural bristle brush, and then brushing your hair completely from roots to ends.

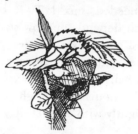

LOTION TO SOOTHE A BALD HEAD

After you shave your head, apply a soothing decoction of any of the following herbs or combinations of herbs: Maidenhair Fern, Wormwood, Southernwood, Sage, Wood Betony, Vervain, Marjoram, Myrtle, Nettle, Rosemary, Rose, Dill, Fennel, or Mistletoe.

BEVERAGE TEA FOR HAIR HEALTH

Healthy hair needs such things as lecithin, vitamin A, vitamin E, and vitamin D, tryptophane, methionine, vegetable oil, biotin, PABA, folic acid, pantothenic acid, copper, and zinc added to the diet. You can mix an herbal tea that contains many of these natural substances as follows:

1 oz. Jamaica flowers	1 oz. Violet leaves
1 oz. Peppermint leaf	1 oz. Dulse
1 oz. Elder blossoms	1 oz. Parsley
1 oz. Lemongrass	1 oz. Rosemary
1 oz. Dandelion	1 oz. Fenugreek seeds, bruised

Mix the herbs together. Store away in a cool, dark place.

When needed, pour 1 cup of boiling water over 1 T.–1 oz. of the herbs in a teapot. Infuse for 3–10 minutes, depending on the strength you prefer. Drink 1–4 cups/day over an extended period of time.

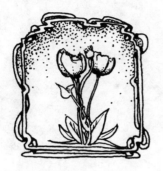

Chapter XVII

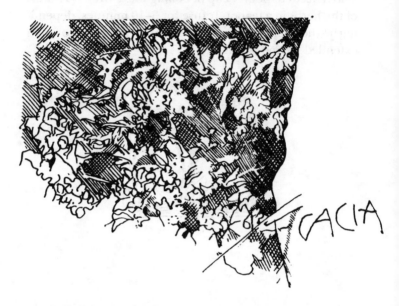

ACACIA

Natural Dyes and Rinses

BASIC DYE RECIPE

TAKE 1–4 oz. of powdered herbs, depending on the length of your hair, and put them into a nonmetal or earthen pot with 2 cups of water. If this isn't enough water to cover the herbs, then add more! You will want enough water to make a thick pack, but not enough to make a thin rinse. Now bring your herbs and water to a boil over a water bath.[1] Immediately remove from heat *or* simmer for a few minutes.

    1. First wash the hair with a good quality castile shampoo, rinse with clear hot water, and towel dry.

[1]Water bath: a pot that contains water in which you place another pot with herbs to heat. Functions about the same as a double boiler.

2. Apply a thick layer of grease or lanolin to the hairline so as not to dye your skin.

3. Wearing rubber gloves and after the thick herby mess cools enough to touch, apply it while still warm to your moistly dry, sectioned hair, starting from the roots and working only one section at a time, applying the pack evenly and on both sides of the section.

4. Then sweep the glucky stuff up into the hair, completely saturating each strand, and then roll the hair up and flat to the head.

5. A roll of cotton or thick roll of toilet paper goes around the hair line to keep the pack from dripping onto the skin.

6. Wrap your head in a muslin cloth or cotton dishtowel wrung out in hot water.

7. Cover your head tightly with a plastic bag or cap to keep the head warm and the herbs working. The herbs stop working as soon as they cool. You can also sit under a warm dryer, wrap your head in hot towels, or stand in front of a warm heater.

8. Allow the paste to stay on the hair for 5 minutes to 12 hours, depending on the color of your hair and depending on the shade you desire. I have very dark hair and let Henna pack stay on my hair over 3 hours each time I do it. Other dark-haired girls allow Henna to stay 4 or 5 hours; Debbie, who has red hair already, leaves Henna on only 20 minutes, and a blond friend allows her weekly Camomile pack only 15 minutes to do its work. So check the color periodically and stop when the desired shade is reached. Since Henna does not really develop until the next day I suggest you allow a dye pack to stay 10 minutes maximum the first week you use it and increase the time week by week until you know exactly how long it takes for

your particular hair to change color with natural dyes.

9. After the color has developed, rinse the hair over and over again with hot water, wearing rubber gloves, until the herbs are completely removed, and the water rinses clean. Then rinse with COLD water to close the pores.

10. Towel dry your hair and brush it when completely dry. Some herbal dye packs are rather astringent and should be followed by an herbal conditioning rinse.

WHAT HERBS TO USE TO DYE OR COLOR THE HAIR

Henna (cements split ends)—reddish hair; Henna and Cloves—dark red brown; Henna and Logwood—deep reddish brown; Sage and Cloves—brownish; Henna and Indigo—blackish brown; Walnut hulls—dark brown; Sage and borax—darken gray hair; Tag Alder bark—gray hair; Black or Blue Malva—blue to blond or white hair; Rosemary, Elder, and borax—brighten brown hair; Golden Seal and Gold Thread—brighten yellow hair; Camomile, Lemon peel, and Marigold—condition and lighten brown hair and brighten and lighten blond hair; Camomile and Quassia—brighten mousy blond hair; Rosemary and Southernwood—brighten dull dark hair; Alkanet and Henna—red hair; Henna and Camomile—golden red color; Rhubarb root developed in the sun gives hair a golden color.

This is just a sample of the colors you can obtain; experiment with the herbs and your hair, because the final color cannot be predicted. Color develops over a period of weeks in most cases and looks brighter in the sunlight. Herbal dyes are especially good for thin hair because they add body, for limp hair because they improve the texture, and for lackluster hair because they bring out the sheen and luster of hair. Most are usually not good for gray hair, and the colors are unpredictable on chemically dyed hair or hair with chemicals in it.

BASIC COLORING RINSE RECIPE

Take 1–4 heaping T. of powdered herbs, depending on the length of your hair and the depth of color you desire (time and practice will tell), put them into a small nonmetal pot and add 2 cups of water. Bring to a boil and *simmer* for 10–20 minutes. Take off the heat and infuse until cool enough to use. Strain.

1. First wash the hair with an herbal castile shampoo that incorporates the same herbs as those you will rinse with, or with any other castile shampoo. Rinse with clear water and towel dry until damp.
2. Wrap a roll of cotton around the hair line to keep the rinse from dripping onto your face.
3. Pour the strained infusion through your hair and into a basin, pour and repour many times rubbing it onto the roots until your hair is completely wet. Wring out the excess.
4. Rinse lightly but completely and towel dry. For light-colored shades it helps to let the sun dry your hair, running your fingers through the strands until it is dry. Dark hair is better dried indoors.

The natural dye herbs are the same as the herbs used for a coloring rinse, the only difference being that you use a larger quantity of herbs or more concentrated herb mixtures for a longer time when dyeing and less quantity, less concentrated when color rinsing.

TO DARKEN THE HAIR

Make a thick decoction of any of these herbs in water, wine, or vinegar: Grape leaves, Willow bark, Walnut bark and hulls, Pomegranate bark, Artichoke leaves, Catechu, Mulberry leaves, Fig leaves, Raspberry leaves, Logwood, Bean shells, Myrtle leaves, Ivy berries and Poppy flowers. The decoction can be made in an iron pot with the addition of a cephalic plant such as: Sage, Marjoram, Balm, Betony, or Laurel.

Henna is a terrific rinse for the hair because it gives reflections.

TO REDDEN THE HAIR

Make a thick decoction of any of the following herbs according to the basic recipes: Radish, Henna, Privet, Birch bark, Saffron, or Marigold.

TO DARKEN THE HAIR OR BEARD AFTER IT HAS BEEN SHAVED

> 1½ oz. oil of Costus
> 1½ oz. oil of Myrtle

Mix these in a lead or iron mortar and then add:

> ½ oz. liquid Pitch, ½ oz. Walnut leaf juice, ½ oz. Laudanum
> 1 drachm Gall nuts, Black-lead, and Frankincense
> a sufficient quantity of mucilage of Gum Arabic made with decoction of Gall nuts

This is another old recipe from the *Toilet* but might be dangerous to use because of the addition of lead.

HERBS TO LIGHTEN HAIR

Frequently wash the hair with the decoction of the herbs and brush through your hair every day an infusion of: Turmeric, Saffron, Yellow Mullein flowers, Yellow Stoechas, Broom, or St. Johnswort.

#36: TO MAKE HAIR OF A FAIR YELLOW GOLDEN COLOR

. . . Or else the haire first clean washed, and then moistened a pretty while by a good fire in warme Allome water with a sponge, you may moisten the same in a decoction of Tumerick, Rubarb, or the Bark of the Barberry tree and so it will receive a most faire and beautiful colour. . . .

—*Delightes for Ladies*

TO TURN GRAY HAIR DARK

Flowers of sulphur rubbed onto the scalp and hair over a few weeks' time will darken it as will a thick decoction of Sage; castor oil; oil of tartar; Tag alder; Artichoke, Raspberry, green shells of Walnut, and Gall, or Bean shells.

Chapter XVIII

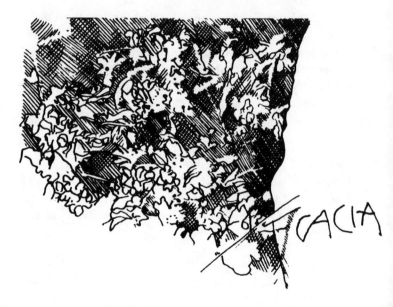

ACACIA

Oil Treatments
and Conditioning Packs

OIL TREATMENTS ARE occasionally necessary to condition a
dry scalp, dry split ends, or damaged hair. They are somewhat difficult to apply and, therefore, a good friend can be
very helpful in assisting.

BASIC OIL TREATMENT DIRECTIONS

1. Brush your hair thoroughly to get rid of loose dirt
   and grime.
2. Wet the hair with warm water so that the oil will be
   mainly absorbed by the scalp rather than the hair.

3. A head steaming will facilitate the absorption of the oil into the scalp.
4. Heat your *oil treatment* slightly, section the hair in areas, and apply the oil treatment to the scalp only, rubbing and massaging it gently onto all areas of the scalp. Pin your hair up in huge pincurls.
5. Wrap your head in a hot towel wrung out in an herbal decoction.
6. Put on a shower cap or wrap your head in hot towels and a plastic bag and keep them hot for a period of 1–4 hours. You could also go under a hair dryer with a hood and set the heat on *warm*.
7. Shampoo with a castile shampoo, rinse completely, shampoo again, and add the juice of ½ Lemon to the shampoo. Rinse, with warm, then hot, then cool water to close the pores.

HERBAL STEAM FOR THE HEAD

A simple mixture, very efficacious for the head, is a mixture of Licorice root, Comfrey leaf, and Violet leaf. Apply according to page 286. Other mixtures such as those listed in Chapter VII can also be used.

HERBAL OIL TREATMENT

Mix together Olive oil, Walnut oil, and peanut oil in equal proportions; to 6 oz. of the mixed oil add ½ oz. Rosemary oil, a few drops of Oregano oil, and Nutmeg oil. Apply about 1 oz. or less to short hair and 1 oz. or more to long hair according to the Basic Oil Treatment Directions.

MORE POTENT HERBAL OIL TREATMENT

A more potent treatment can be made by first infusing herbs in the oils. Mix your Olive and peanut oil. Take 4 oz.

of herbs such as Rosemary, Comfrey, Fennel, and Burdock, and pour over them 2 cups of the oil. *Simmer* in a nonmetal pot until the herbs are crisp, strain out the herbs, and add up to ½ oz. essential oil to 6 oz. of the herbed oil, and proceed according to the Basic Oil Treatment Directions. Essential oils in this case can be *pure* oil of Rosemary or Basil.

AVOCADO SCALP PACK FOR DRY, SUNBURNED, AND OVERBLEACHED HAIR

1. Beat an egg to a froth in a blender and add ½ Avocado until well blended.
2. Apply the green goo, section by section, to your hair, applying from the scalp outward until you reach the end of each strand of hair.
3. Massage completely into the scalp and put on a plastic shower cap, so that the heat from the head will facilitate the absorption of the protein and oils.
4. After 20 minutes, start rinsing off the mixture beginning with cool water, then tepid, and then warm. Never rinse an egg mixture with hot water as it will "cook" and become like scrambled eggs.
5. Rub your hair dry with a towel or with your hands or with a piece of silk for a glossy finish. Then brush.

WILLIAM'S CONDITIONING TREATMENT

1. Brush the hair with a mixture of 2 oz. Olive oil mixed with 2 oz. Rosemary or Lavender oil. Wrap in a scarf wrung out in hot Rosemary infusion. Cover with a shower cap. Leave this on for a few hours or overnight.
2. Separate a couple of eggs and beat the yolks until light and frothy.
3. Wash your hair with the egg yolk, working up the

froth and working it all through the hair. Rinse with tepid water several times.

4. Beat the white with some Lemon juice until frothy and forming light peaks. Now wash the hair with the egg whites, continually working it through the hair. Rinse with tepid water, warm water, Rosemary infusion, and finally a cold rinse.

This is an absolutely fantastic conditioner for all types of hair and can be used weekly.

FOR DAMAGED HAIR

Mix together completely 2 oz. unsweetened condensed milk, 1 T. wheat germ oil, and 1 oz. thick decoction of Cherry bark. Apply according to the Basic Directions.

Some *protein shampoos* coat the hair, can make it *look* healthier, but also coat the scalp, strangling the pores and leaving the scalp scaly and flaky. Herbal shampoos and rinses condition the skin of the scalp, and in time normalize the hair and scalp.

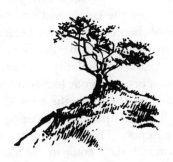

AVOCADO MAYONNAISE OIL TREATMENT CONDITIONER

1. To ½ cup health food, salt-free mayonnaise that

has been made with real eggs and pure Safflower
or Soy oil, add ½ Avocado. Blend together in your
blender.

2. Wet your hair. Apply the Avocado mayonnaise to
the saclp *only*, pinning the hair in big pincurls.
Wrap your head either in an old silk scarf or in a
linen towel wrung out in hot Comfrey leaf or Nettle
or Rosemary water. Then cover it all up with a
plastic shower cap. Wear this for several hours.

3. Rinse your hair with cool, then tepid, then warm
water. Shampoo lightly with an herbal shampoo.
Rinse and rinse with warm water, then cool water.

4. To complete the conditioning, follow with a rinsing of the herbal waters you used in step 2.

JULIANNA'S FATHER'S HAIR RECIPE
TO RETAIN COLOR AND SCALP HEALTH

Get 4 pounds of marrow bones sliced 1 inch thick and
scrape out the marrow. Cut a peeled Potato into large
pieces and place the Potato and the marrow all together in
a small covered enamel pot and cook slowly over low heat
for many hours until the Potato is soft. Julianna says the
smell is lousy. Remove the Potato and strain the substance
through 3 layers of cheesecloth 5 times. Let it rest until cool
but still liquid, add pure oil of Bergamot or Lemon oil to
smell. Seal the jar and let it solidify. It is very oily. When
needed, warm a bit between your hands and work into the
scalp thoroughly and then into the hair. Go about your
business for 2–8 hours and then shampoo with a good
herbal castile shampoo. This is said to be an old Greek
formula to retain rich dark color in the hair.

Chapter XIX

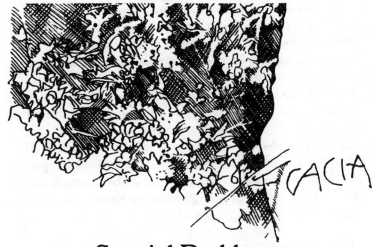

Special Problems:

Dandruff, Brushing, Tangling, How to Curl, How to Straighten, Electricity, Growth, and Baldness

PROPER DIET, REST, AND exercise will go far to alleviate these conditions and a once a month treatment for the hair will pamper it to perfection.

A TREATMENT FOR THE HAIR

When the problems are varied such as hair loss, oiliness of the hair, dandruff, and a dry scalp, or for a once a month treatment for healthy hair—treat your head as gently as you treat your face—steam clean it and occasionally apply medicating masks. Problem hair is often a result of tension and stress, a poor diet, and poor circulation.

Start with an invigorating aroma massage of the shoulder and neck area. Use a Jasmine or Rose base to relax, increase blood circulation, and to relieve tension. Steam clean your scalp by first brushing your hair, then applying a thick infusion of herbs such as Fennel, Rose, and Comfrey to the scalp, thoroughly wetting the hair. Wrap it up in a shower cap. You could take a bath or just relax around the house. This steaming will open and medicate the pores. Now shampoo the hair or apply one of the oil treatments. In any case end up with an herbal shampoo that complements the herbs you used in the steaming and follow it up with a cleansing astringent rinse to close the pores. Remember to rinse and rinse.

To Grow Long Hair, let your bangs grow out. Your body tries to maintain an intimate balance, and if you have short bangs your longer hair will fall out to try to get shorter and your short hair will strive to get longer. In any case the overall result is shorter, thinner hair. The length and strength of the hair depends on the size and strength of the root—the shorter the hair, the smaller and weaker the root and conversely, the longer the hair, the bigger and thicker the root. So if your hair is falling out or splitting, it doesn't make sense to cut it to strengthen it. Condition it to stop the falling out and get an expert to give you a singe cut to seal the split ends. Do not wear rubber bands in your hair, either coated or uncoated. The rubber insulates the hair and stops the normal flow of static electricity—hair elasticity is reduced and it will break more easily. Cleanliness is important as well as a regular brushing with a boar bristle brush.

A TREATMENT FOR FALLING HAIR

Pour 1 qt. of boiling water over 1 oz. of Rosemary leaf, 1 T. baking soda (to soften the water), and 1½ t. Camphor. Let it stand overnight and then strain. Add 4 oz. 50 per cent alcohol (100-proof vodka will do). Apply carefully to the roots of the hair every other day.

TO CURL HAIR AND STIMULATE GROWTH

Mix 1 cup Olive oil with 1 t. oil of Marjoram and add 1 t. oil of Rosemary and rub into the roots daily. This oil is very oily, and I prefer a mixture of equal quantities of Olive oil, Marjoram, and Rosemary.

TO PREVENT BALDNESS AND QUICKEN GROWTH

Powder some Parsley seeds in a seed grinder and powder your head and scalp at night every 3 or 4 months. Dip your comb into Nettle juice and comb your hair every morning lightly in the wrong direction. You can also use Jaborandi water or the juice from the Rosemary or the Southernwood or young Hemp tops infused in water for 24 hours.

#13: A COMPOUND OIL TO QUICKEN GROWTH

Take a pound of green Southernwood bruised, boil it in a pint and a half of Sweet Oil, and a half a pint of Red Wine; when sufficient boiled remove it from the fire, and strain off the liquor through a linen bag: repeat this operation three times with fresh Southernwood. The last time add to the strained liquor 2 oz. of Bears-grease.

This oil quickly makes the hair shoot out.

—*The Toilet of Flora*, 1779

Bear's grease has a long reputation in Europe and with the American Indians as a hair growth stimulator.

TO THICKEN HAIR AND TO STIMULATE GROWTH

    2 oz. Maidenhair root
    2 oz. Cabbage leaves and cores
    2 oz. Hemp root

Dry the herbs and burn them; make a lye of the ashes and wash the head with the lye for 3 days in succession, firstly rubbing the head with pure honey.

This is an adaptation from an old recipe and as I have never used it I cannot speak of its efficacy.

AN OLD FORMULA TO MAKE HAIR GROW IN A BALD PART AND TO THICKEN THE HAIR

Melt together ¼ lb. each of chicken fat, Hempseed oil, and honey in a pot, take off the heat, and stir with a wooden spoon until cold. You must apply this cream on the indicated place for 8 days in succession.

A GROWTH STIMULATOR

Brush your hair daily with oil of Rosemary, oil of Lavender, or oil of Basil, or a mixture thereof; rub a lotion of the following into the hair every night: 1 oz. Olive or Walnut oil shaken with 1 oz. Rosemary oil and 8 drops of oil of Nutmeg.

Even though Walnut oil is used in some recipes to stimulate growth it also appears in other recipes to prevent growth, such as this recipe listed in *The Toilet of Flora*. Oil of Walnuts, frequently rubbed on a child's forehead, will prevent the hair from growing on that part.

A GROWTH STIMULATOR #2

Macerate Peach kernels with a pestle and pour over 1 oz. of this maceration 4 oz. of boiling Apple cider vinegar. Infuse for 9 days, shaking the container daily. Rub this into the scalp daily.

Scaly Scalp—Seborrhea Dermatitis (Dandruff)
Symptoms are dry scalp, over-oily hair. Hair root is inflamed, and the oil glands are overactive. Stress and our synthetic diet are often causes. The cure is Lemongrass rinse or any of the herbal rinses for dandruff.

SCALY SCALP FOODS

Stay away from starches, spicy foods, and alcohol. Increase vitamin B, cheese, nuts, eggs, green vegetables, fruits, skim milk, lean meat, and fish.

DANDRUFF

Dandruff often occurs in people with unusually oily skin and scalp, a result of a dysfunction of the sebaceous, or oil-producing, glands in skin and scalp. Dandruff *itches*—while scaly scalp doesn't—and it results from poor diet, endocrine imbalance, and emotional stress. Treatment is tar and herbal shampoos. Dandruff heads should rinse, rinse, rinse, with cool water—oily hairs use water and vinegar, a modern as well as old cure for oily hair, and add borax as a softener to rinse water. Keep hair spray to a minimum. Avoid hot hair dryers. Don't tint or permanent; both of these are damaging. Bathe scalp in hot herbal oils. Dry hairs, shampoo less frequently and condition with herbal rinse.

FOR DANDRUFF

Make a very thick decoction of White Willow or Birch bark. Mix 1 oz. of the strained decoction with 1 oz. of your favorite herbal shampoo. Shampoo as usual with the mixture and rinse with the herbal solution, pouring and repouring through the hair, and concentrating on the scalp. You may give it a final rinse with cool water to close the pores.

TO REMOVE DANDRUFF

Add borax to Rosemary water and comb the hair backwards with this solution daily, concentrating on the scalp. Backcombing is not very good for the hair; an alternate solution to get the boraxed Rosemary water to the scalp would be to dip your fingerpads into the liquid and rub onto the scalp in vigorous circular, small, zigzag motions.

HERBAL HAIR RINSE FOR DANDRUFF

This mixture of herbs is useful as either a vinegar rinse or an herbal infusion.

1. Mix equal quantities of medicating herbs such as White Willow bark, Quassia chip, Bergamot (or Creosote).
2. Mix equal quantities of stimulating herbs such as Nettle, Arnica, or Peppermint leaves.
3. Mix 2 oz. of the medicating herbs with 1 oz. of the stimulating herbs.

Now you may either rinse your hair with an herbal infusion according to the basic directions in Chapter XVI or you can make a vinegar conditioning rinse as follows: Pour 1 cup boiling Apple cider vinegar over 1 oz. of the mixed herbs. Infuse over a week's time, shaking the container daily. Strain out the herbs and use 1 T.–¼ cup of the Herbal Vinegar to 1 cup of water when you rinse your hair after a shampoo. You may also use the Herbal Vinegar or the Herbal Infusion daily to treat the dandruff by rubbing it into the scalp.

DANDRUFF TREATMENT

1. Make sure that your diet is right.
2. Make the dandruff shampoo according to Chapter XV and use.
3. Apply the dandruff rinse according to Chapter XVI or as above.
4. Every 10 days to 2 weeks apply one of the oil treatments.
5. Be persistent in your treatments.

BRUSHING

The importance of proper brushing with a natural boar bristle brush cannot be overemphasized. It stimulates the scalp, distributes the natural oils, removes the daily accumulation of dust, lint, and air pollutants, improves elasticity, and gives the hair body and strength. The correct brushing procedure for both males and females is this: Jump out of bed in the morning. Stand with feet planted firmly on the floor, bend over at the waist until the head is parallel to the knees and let hair hang down. In this position, brush hair with one hand and stroke the brushed hair with the other palm. Brush from the nape of the neck to the ends. This upside down brushing massages the scalp properly and completely. (In standing up brushing tension is caused when you lift your elbows above the shoulders, restricting blood flow to the scalp.) Proper brushing will also distribute the natural oils from the new hair at the nape of the oil-poor hair at the ends. And furthermore, the open-palm strokes will counteract static electricity build-up.

CLEANSING HAIRBRUSHES AND COMBS

It would be wise to invest in a hairbrush brush and a comb brush. Never wash your combs and brushes in soap and hot water as the soap softens the bristles, and the hot water further destroys them. Pull out all loose hairs from the brush with the hairbrush brush. Dissolve 1 tablespoon of ordinary baking soda or hydrogen peroxide solution in cool water and drop in your brushes and combs. Swish them around, brush the comb with the comb brush from the top down through the teeth to remove all the impurities. Brush the brush with the hairbrush; brush from the back to the ends of the bristles. Rinse in cool water and set aside to dry on a terry towel, bristles of the brush down so that the water does not drain into the handle or the back.

TO CLEAN THE HAIR AND HAIRBRUSHES AND COMBS

Dissolve 1 oz. borax and ½ oz. Camphor in a quart of boiling water. Let the solution cool. Drop in the combs and brushes (cleaned of hair). Swish them around a lot, shake them out, rinse in warm water and drain, bristle-side down on a linen or terry towel. This solution is also good as a rinse for the hair to cleanse and strengthen it.

TO CLEAN WOODEN COMBS

Brush out debris with a brush especially made for combs. Apply oil to the comb and brush it out. If you have a wooden comb and are married, don't throw it out—the

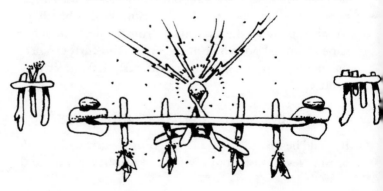

Japanese say that if you do, you mean to throw out the marriage (get a divorce).

FOR STATIC ELECTRICITY BUILD-UP

When you brush your hair follow each stroke of the brush with your other hand, palm open.

HAIR SETTING LOTIONS

1. ¼ oz. Irish Moss boiled in 1 qt. of water until it is a mucilage. Bottle in 8 oz. wide-mouthed bottles with 1 T. of alcohol as a preservative. Dip the comb in the bottle and set the hair as usual.
2. Mucilage of Tragacanth scented with any essence. This won't keep and should be freshly made each time you set your hair. To make, soak 1½ t. of Tragacanth in 1 cup of water or Rosemary water for 24 hours.

SEAWEED HAIR SET

2 T. Irish Moss	2 T. bay rum
1 qt. infusion of Rosemary or Lavender water	1 t. Rosemary or Lavender oil

Simmer Irish Moss in the Rosemary water for about 1 hour. Wring through muslin and add the bay rum and scent.

HAIR SLICKER/HAIR SETTER

1 oz. gum Tragacanth
2¾ cups Rosewater
a few drops of oil of Rose or any other scent
    you like (optional)

Steep the gum in the Rosewater for a day or two. Shake frequently while it forms a mucilage. After about 2 days, strain through absolutely clean, coarse linen. You can let it stand for a few days more and strain again, but in any case, when it forms a uniform consistency, add the oil and use either to set your hair, or to train it into position.

The Rosewater may be colored with Alkanet, or Blue Malva, or Parsley, or Jamaica flowers by adding ½ oz. to the Rosewater and letting it sit for a day, straining out the herb, and then adding to the Tragacanth to form the mucilage.

TO CURL OR SET THE HAIR

Brush your hair with a mucilage of Iceland Moss, Gum Arabic, Quince seed, Flax seed, or wash with Rosemary infusion. (To make a mucilage see Chapter II.)

TO CURL OILY HAIR

Boil 2 cups of water and 1 T. of Quince seed until you have about 1 cup. Strain and add 3 oz. alcohol or your favorite cologne. Brush into the hair or use as a setting lotion.

HAIR TOO CURLY

Iron[1] it with a flat iron, set on cool, and then condition it. Groom with a light hair cream or a growth stimulator. No hair spray.

TO STRAIGHTEN HAIR

Soak Alkanet in Vaseline until it is pink, strain out the Alkanet, add tincture of Benzoin, 2 drops per ounce, and oil of Bergamot or oil of Citronella. Brush into the hair every day.

---

[1]Lay your hair out on an ironing board and have a friend iron your hair with a cool iron, being careful to iron only the hair and not the head. I used to iron Patty's hair this way after each shampooing.

B IS FOR BODY

Treat your body as well as you treat your face and it will reward you with increased vigor and vitality.

Bathe it in herbs, powder it soft and smooth, bathe and massage with aromatic oils, protect it from fat and the hot sun, pet it, nurture it, and feed it well—not abundantly, but well.

As Ms. Leyel has said, ". . . LIVING HERBS—living, because unlike drugs, they are organic and not inorganic. They are natural food and medicine for the membranes, glands and tissues. . . ."

—*The Truth About Herbs,* 1943

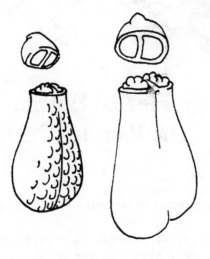

Chapter XX

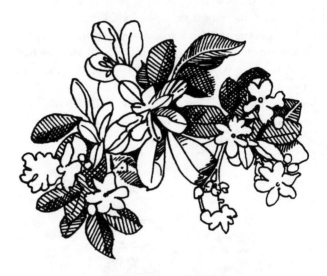

Herbal Baths,
the Wonder Cure

. . . Ah, the sybaritic pleasures of an outdoor bath . . .

A BEAUTIFUL BODY is primarily the result of the right diet, healthy invigorating exercise, regular rest, and cleanliness. Herbal baths are the organic antidote to impure air and harsh water conditions. Herbal baths using only unsprayed herbs are for smoothing, soothing, and hydrating the skin, to keep it healthy and young looking. They should be taken by both men and women at least 2–3 times per week. Indeed, there are several ways to take an herbal bath or shower:

BASIC BATH RECIPES

1. Place a large handful or about ½ cupful of herbs in a covered nonmetal pot and add water to cover. Bring to a boil and *simmer* the contents for 10–20 minutes to extract all the wonderful beneficial contents of the herbs. Strain the material, use the herbs as a scrub and pour the liquid into your tub, or use the liquid as a last rinse when you shower. If you are bathing, try to soak in the herbal extracts for at least 20 minutes.

2. Buy a metal or, preferably an enamel or china, rice cooking ball in the kitchen specialty department of your favorite store. Half fill it with herbs and pop into your tub. They usually have a chain attached with a hook that you can hook onto your faucet so the water of the shower or tub can run through. This is by far the easiest way to take an herbal bath or shower.

3. Wrap a large handful of herbs in a washcloth and tie with a string. Drop into a pot of boiling water to extract the essence and then dump the whole thing into your tub or make a bath bag of muslin with a

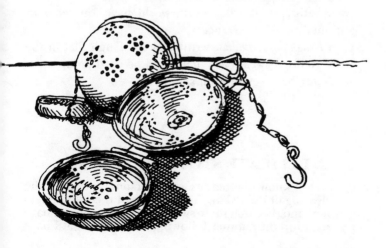

drawstring top. Scrub with the bath bag and rinse
with the liquid.
4. Pop a handful of herbs directly into your bath,
soak, and enjoy. (Careful, it might clog your drain
temporarily.)

After all, our skin is the largest organ of the body and
one of the organs of excretion. It is made of two layers
called the dermis and the epidermis. The top layer or
epidermis is made up of nice plump cells that divide to
form new cells that come to the surface of the epidermis
and harden and is then called keratin, a type of protein.
This dead protein layer is removed by washing or exfoliation and if not removed, it combines with oil and bacteria
that grows on it to become that dreadful moneymaker *body
odor*. Under the epidermis is the dermis which is composed
of hair roots, blood vessels, nerve endings, and the glands
that produce sebum (oil) and sweat. And underneath all of
this is fat. Between these three layers are the muscle fibers
and connective tissue that hold it all together and keep the
skin flexible, strong, and elastic.

Sweat is one of the best ways of cleansing the body and
sweat baths, popular all over the world, have both religious
and medicinal importance.

In *Delightes for Ladies*, written by Sir Hugh Plat in the
early 1600s, a sweat bath that could be used today is described. I have rewritten it slightly:

A DELICATE STOVE TO SWEAT IN

. . . I know that many Gentlepersons, as well for the
clearing of their skins, as cleansing of their bodies, do
now and then delight to sweat. For this purpose, I have
set down the manner following, as the best that I have

ever observed: Put into a large brass pot, sweat herbs of a kind that are most appropriate for your infirmity, with a reasonable quantity of water; close the pot tightly with a well-fitting top; at some part of the cover you must let in a pipe (the entrance whereof must be conveyed through the side of the chimney), where the pot stands in a thick hollow stake of a bathing tub crossed with hoops, according to the usual manner, in the top, which you may cover with a sheet at your pleasure. Now, the steam of the pot passing through the pipe under the half bottom of the bathing tub, which must be bored full of big holes, will breathe so sweet and warm a vapour upon your body, (as that receiving air, by holding your head without the tub as you sit within it) you shall sweat, and continue so without fainting. And this is performed with a small charcoal fire maintained under the pot for this purpose. Note, that the room would be closed where you place your bathing tub, lest any sudden cold should happen to offend you whilst your body is made open and porous to the air. . . .

Another way to take a steam bath without having a steam room is described in *My Water-Cure*, by Sebastian Kneipp. Get a very large pail and place over it a chair with no seat. Put herbs into the pail and fill with furiously boiling water. Immediately sit on the chair—naked of course—and cover yourself and the chair with a large woolen blanket or a plastic sheet, held tightly around the neck so that no steam escapes. Sit there until no more steam rises and you start to cool. Then either have someone else replace the water with more boiling water or wrap yourself in an enormous towel and towel dry. I prefer to sit in the steam tent and wipe off the sweat with hand towels as it occurs, and to continue steaming until the pores are completely open and clean. Then I either shower or jump into a warm herb tub, wrap in a towel, and air dry rather than towel dry.

There are baths for every purpose. Use Chapter I to decide which herbs for what purpose you want to pop into the bath with you.

NINON'S FAVORITE REJUVENATING AND
REGENERATING HERBS

This is my favorite bath and after having used at least several hundred different bath herb mixtures, this is the one I keep coming back to. If used often enough it will smooth and help maintain the normal fluid content of your skin—thereby keeping it firm and young looking.

1 oz. Lavender	1 oz. Lemon Thyme
1 oz. Rosemary	1 oz. fresh or dried Roses
1 oz. Peppermint	1 oz. Houseleek or Aloe
1 oz. Comfrey root	

The Lavender is for acne and to reduce puffiness; the Rosemary to regain energy and do away with evil, is astringent and diaphoretic; the Peppermint is a stimulating, cooling aromatic; the Comfrey contains allantoin, is healing, regenerative and an emollient; the Lemon Thyme is an antiseptic, local anesthetic, and mild deodorant; the Roses are used as a hydrater; and the Houseleek or Aloe as a cooling astringent for any kind of skin problems.

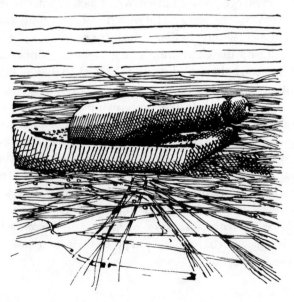

PARCHMENT SKIN BATH FOR REJUVENATING AND REGENERATING

Mix together equal parts of Patchouli, Savory, Vetivert, Linden, Sandalwood, and Comfrey leaf.

This mixture is expecially favored by men. First, spray a bit of oil of Patchouli on the Patchouli herb. Mix it well and then combine the Patchouli with the rest of the herbs. Use about 4 oz. for a really efficacious bath. The Patchouli has a rejuvenating effect on the senses, Savory for stimulating, Vetivert is a tonic stimulant, Sandalwood in conjunction with Vetivert is beneficial to healthy skin tone and for inflammations, and Comfrey regenerates aging skin.

LOVE BATH

Make a cold infusion of Honeysuckle, Jasmine, Acacia, Fuchsia, and Carnation. After a few hours drop this into your bath along with a hot infusion of Red Clover, Deer Tongue, and Orange peel. Take a long soaking bath; this will leave a wonderful aromatic scent on your skin and is wonderful to take with a friend.

STIMULATING WAKE-UP BATH

Mike and I have been experimenting for some time with mixtures of herbs that would stimulate one's senses in the mornings when we usually are exhausted and can't keep our eyes open. One day I dropped a very large handful of Nettle into his tub while he was resting against the edge. The Nettles got caught in the space between the tub and his back. Everything was all right until he got up to dry off when we noticed a large red and slightly blistered area on his back which itched like crazy. After applying about a pound of thick salve, and Bruise Juice,[1] the itch finally subsided and some days later the redness finally left too. It

[1]See *Herbs & Things*, p. 204.

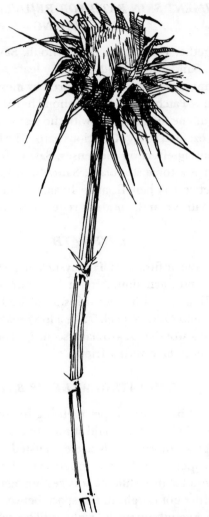

goes without saying that a Nettle bath is indeed stimulating but should definitely *not* be added directly to the tub. Always make this bath in a pot, pour the liquid into the tub, and wrap the herbs in a cloth or use any of the first three basic bath recipes.

Mix equal quantities of Nettle, Rosemary, Lemon balm,

Savory, Lavender, and Comfrey leaf. Add scented Geranium if you have it.

SIMPLE BATH

Simple bath mixtures are also very nice. Linden (Tilia or Lime) blossoms, added to the bath, act as a sedative and are very soothing and mildly diaphoretic; Lavender is wonderfully stimulating; Houseleek is used for its healing powers; Peppermint containing menthol is cooling and aromatic; Yarrow is a potent astringent.

MUSCLE-RELAXING BATH

2 oz. Sassafras bark	1 oz. Agrimony
1 oz. Burdock root	1 oz. Comfrey leaf
1 oz. Mugwort	1 oz. Sage

This bath is formulated to help relax sore, tired, and strained muscles and for muscular aches and pains.

SERENITY BATH

a large handful of Violet leaves for vitamin C
a large handful of Pansies for salicylic acid
a large handful of Cowslips, Spearmint, and Roses
a small handful of Mistletoe herb

This is an old mixture that was used by the ancient herbalists to ease melancholy, invoke tenderness, and the scent was thought to draw the mind into quieter passageways. Add a spray of essence of Violets for a more potent effect. Other tranquilizing herbs are Passionflower, Vervain, Camomile, Sage, St. Johnswort, Peach leaf, Burdock, Meadowsweet, or Balm.

FLORA'S NO. 1 BATH

Simmer in a pot for some minutes in spring water some of

the following herbs: Laurel, Thyme, Rosemary, Marjoram, Lavender, Southernwood, Wormwood, Sage, Pennyroyal, Sweet Basil, Balm, Mint, Hyssop, Anise, Fennel, or any other herb that smells good.

This is a terrific bath, said to strengthen the legs and arms, is diaphoretic, and relieves pain that comes from being cold.

BARLEY BATH TO CLEANSE AND SOFTEN THE SKIN

Mix together 1 lb. Barley, 4 lb. Bran and 8 oz. Borage flowers and leaves; boil them in a quantity of water until everything is soft and mushy. Strain the liquid into the tub, wrap the solid matter in cheesecloth.

You needn't use soap with this bath; it is sufficient to scrub your skin with the Barley bag.

SUPER CLEANSING BATH

Start a hot bath and add 1 lb. of Epsom salts and 1 lb. of Bay salt. Sit in the tub up to your neck for 45 minutes, no more and no less. This is the time needed to fully open your pores and bring the impurities to the surface. Take a muslin bag filled with salt and rub your body, one leg at a time from the toes up to the groin and from the head down to the groin. Do this quickly in circular motions. Now rinse your body in the tub to get rid of waste and toxins that you have brought to the surface. Either take a cleansing warm shower or get out of the tub and towel dry with several small hand towels.

I like to take this bath every couple of months or so, especially when I have been under stress for some time and need a break.

SUMMER BATH FOR COOLING THE ITCH

Run a bath and add about ½ lb. Oatmeal. Stand in the tub

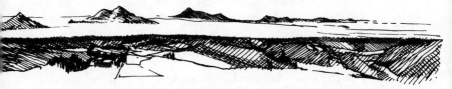

with a handful of Oatmeal and cover your body with it. Scrub with a bristle body brush, a friction strap, or a loofah. Sit in the tub and soak, get out, and *air dry*.

SUPER MILK BATH

It is easy to dump some skim milk powder into a bathtub full of water and take a milk bath, but it's much nicer to increase the power of the milk by adding herbs. For instance, take a large quantity of Camomile flowers and infuse in warm skim milk for some hours. Pour the milk into the tub and put the Camomile flowers into a bag to wash with. Linden, Elder flowers, Jasmine, Honeysuckle, Tuberose, Strawberries, and many other botanicals can be used in this manner.

ROSES AND ORANGES BATH FOR LITTLE CHILDREN

Add handfuls of Roses, Rose leaves, Rose hips, Camomile, Orange flowers, Orange peel, Lemon peel, and Orange leaves to a pot. Let it simmer, pour the liquid into the tub, and scrub with a muslin bag of the herbs.

Children love this bath because it is so colorful and sweetly aromatic.

FOREST BATHS FOR ALL SEASONS

Collect Pine, Fir, or Cedar needles in season. When you wish to relive the refreshing feel of the forest, take your needles and make a decoction. Add Meadowsweet or Marjoram, Melilot or Clover, and pour this mixture into the tub with a drop of Fir essence.

"Ummmmmmmm," Great for the overtired or debilitated senses and very refreshing to the respiratory organs.

HOT AND COLD

For the really fatigued body and to tone up the muscles, take alternating hot and cold baths. Add Pine needles to the hot and Rosemary to the cold: this is very stimulating and refreshing.

LEMONS AND GRAPEFRUITS, STRAWBERRIES AND BLACKBERRIES

Make an infusion of Strawberry and Blackberry leaves, and pour this into the bath. Cut a Lemon and a Grapefruit into thick slices and drop into the tub. Scrub with the berry leaves wrapped in muslin and follow by rubbing your body all over with the Lemon and Grapefruit slices. Great for overly oily skin and as a skin stimulating tonic.

FOR OILY SKIN

Mix Lemongrass, Lemon peels, White Willow bark, Pansies, Peppermint, and Witch Hazel in equal quantities. Make a decoction of 4 oz. of the herbs. Take a shower with soap. Then a *warm* soaking bath containing the decoction. Rub the herbs all over your body. Get out of the tub, wrap loosely in cotton and *drain dry*.

GINSENG DRY SKIN BATH

1 oz. Comfrey root
¼ oz. of Ginseng (buy Ginseng by the pound, it is much cheaper this way and will last for ages)

1 oz. Patchouli
1 oz. Roses sprayed with essence of Rose

Make a decoction of the Comfrey and Ginseng, and an

infusion of the Patchouli and Roses. Mix the two liquids together and add to your bath, or after your shower pat dry your skin and pat the liquid on with a muslin bag containing the herbs.

SWEAT BATH FOR A COLD

A mixture of Borage, Camomile, Elder, Pennyroyal, Burdock, and Marigolds makes an excellent restorative sweat bath when you have a cold.

HEAT RASH BATH

The best bath to take, for an infant or an adult, when you have prickly heat or heat rash is the laundry starch bath. Make Comfrey root decoction. Pour the liquid decoction into a *warm* bath containing about 1 lb. of laundry starch. Both cooling and healing.

SALTWATER BATH

Mix 1 lb. sea salt, ½ lb. powdered Irish Moss, ½ lb. bicarbonate of soda. Spray the whole with oil of Lavender. Whenever you want to be reminded of the sea put about ½ lb. of this mix into your tub. It can be made in larger quantities and stored indefinitely for use. I love it and use it several times a month. Very toning and most refreshing.

SIMPLE BATH HERB RECIPE #2

Mix equal quantities of Sage, Rosemary, Lavender, and Basil and use about 4 oz. per bath.

PRICKLY SKIN BATH

If your skin feels all prickly and sensitive—as it usually does when you have a cold—take a bath of Elder flowers and colloidal Oatmeal.

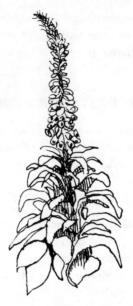

AN HERBAL BATH FOR THE FIVE SENSES

Nine herbs to enliven and enhance the senses: Add Roses or Elder, Melilot, Cowslips, Wintersweet or Meadowsweet, Orris, Cinquefoil, Primrose, Violet leaves, and Buckwheat to your bath. Add essence of Tuberose. Now turn out the lights and let these cleansing, healing herbs to their work, medicating your body by an osmotic influence.

FINALLY, FOR PINEAL POWER

Take a medicating, tranquilizing, hot, soaking, meditating bath, and drink teas of Mugwort, Parsley, Bamboo, Rue, Yarrow, and Borage—all these herbs have a folk history of opening the third eye—Mugwort is also known as an herb that induces or increases clairvoyance (or for curing excessive opium smoking).

Chapter XXI

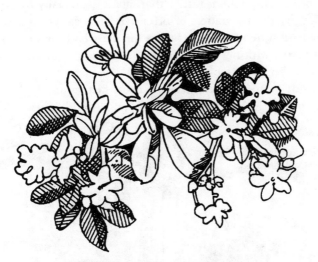

Herbal Powders
and Deodorants

A LITTLE ARTICLE that I cut out from I know not where states, "Sage for Odor Control". "Research on the feeding habits of deer in Colorado may have uncovered an idea for controlling feedlot odors. Scientists are finding that chopped sagebrush added to the diets of fattening steers reduces odors. The additive has no adverse effect on feed efficiency, carcass quality, or taste of the meat. Oils in the sagebrush change the make-up of the bacterial population in the animals' digestive tracts, modifying waste odors."

Could it be that there are actually herbal deodorants? It seems so for cattle, and, fortunately, there are herbal deodorants for humans too. Some of these natural deodorants are eaten to improve one's personal scent, and some of them are used externally to mask the natural body odors; some used externally seem to combine with one's odor to complement rather than mask it—usually by not allowing the formation of offensive bacteria. Of course, the easiest deodorizing agent is the daily bath or shower, especially with herbs that sweeten the body scent and improve the texture of the skin.

Body odors are intensified by many factors not the least of which is the horrible processed, "improved," "enriched"

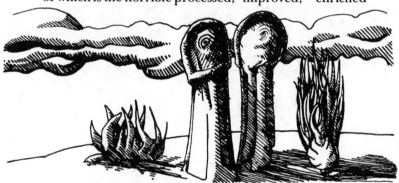

junk that most Americans seem to like to eat. The next most important factor in body odor is synthetic fabrics that coat our bodies with an impermeable layer—impermeable to air that is—that seem to strangle and suffocate our bodies with its own effluvia. They do not permit the skin to breathe. And added to this diet of processed food and synthetic coverings is that even the very air we breathe is loaded with soot and smog which strangle our pores and clog them with impurities.

Some of the foods directly effecting how we smell are meat and vegetables. It seems that a diet high in meat makes for a stronger body odor, and one higher in vegetables than meat has less of an effect on body odor. Eating yogurt consistently has a beneficial effect by changing the bacterial population, and stress and tension have a negative effect. Alcohol has a definite negative effect.

Experiment with what you eat and maybe you too will find that some foods make you smell better than other foods, just as the scientists discovered with the Sagebrush.

As a matter of fact, Sage (a different genus than Sagebrush) has an historical use as a deodorizing tea. And the Mints, especially Peppermint, are especially useful when you are flatulent (use 2 drops in an ounce of water and drink every hour or so).

Besides bathing, some of the more useful and easier to use herbal underarm deodorants are:

1. Witch Hazel leaf or bark decoction or Witch Hazel extract as an underarm splash to remove odor.
2. White Willow bark. An infusion of White Willow bark mixed with borax acts as a deodorant wash for offensive-smelling perspiration. Mix a few drops of oil of Patchouli with the infusion. . . . *Herbs & Things,* 1972.
3. Orange peel mixed with Lemon peel and powdered is a nice underarm deodorizer.
4. Thyme decoction as an after bath splash.
5. Wearing cotton garments is helpful as well as a diet as natural as possible.
6. Chaparral (creosote) decoction externally applied is a natural deodorizer.
7. Rose Astringent Lotion in Chapter X is an excellent underarm deodorant that I use daily.

HERBAL DEODORANT POWDER

Mix together equal quantities of powdered Orris root, Orange peel powder, and Lemon peel powder. Add a bit of powdered Calamus root or Licorice root to scent. Now mix it all together and sift through a fine sifter. Use as a powder under the arms, on the pubic area, or on the body. Anything can cause an allergic reaction and Orris root has often caused reactions, so before trying any herb in quantity, try a little bit first and if you get no reaction then it is probably all right for you to use.

The same goes for commercial deodorants. Many of

them contain highly suspect ingredients and, unfortunately at this time, there is no law in effect that says they have to list the ingredients on their labels. But if you make your own cosmetics you will know what they are being made of and can, therefore, keep out all suspect ingredients or any materials that you are allergic to.

HEXACHLOROPHENE

There are at least two dozen cosmetic products on sale, including deodorants, body powders, baby powders, and vaginal deodorants, in which hexachlorophene is named as an ingredient. Significant quantities of this chemical have also been discovered in several deodorants, cosmetics, and make-up products without any mention on the container. As you probably are aware, this ingredient has been implicated in various abnormalities of the fetus and has also caused severe allergic reactions in the pubic and underarm areas of many adults. Recent scientific tests indicate that chemicals including hexachlorophene enter the body much more rapidly through the sensitive vaginal area. Wouldn't it be safer to wash with soap and water and pat a gentle herbal powder on your baby, your underarms, or your pubic area as a deodorant, rather than using an ingredient that might be harmful to you or your child?

BABY POWDER

  2 oz. pure unscented Montana talcum powder
       (arsenic occurs naturally in association with
       talc, and Montana talc seemingly has the
       least)
  1 oz. Camomile flowers, PO
  1 oz. Calendula flowers, PO

Mix all ingredients and sift through a very fine sieve. Corn starch can be substituted for the talc. This powder is cooling and absorbent and will be effective in treating diaper rash and other skin irritations.

BODY POWDER

Many *powdered* herbs can be effectively used as body powders or deodorant powders; among these are Patchouli, Orris root, Orange peel, Orange flowers, Lemon peel, Calamus root, Licorice root, Sandalwood, Marigold, Camomile, Rose, and Lavender. Some of the darker herbs such as Patchouli and Cornsilk, though helpful for skin irritations, will sometimes stain light colored clothes and probably should be mixed with other powders as a body powder rather than as an underarm powder. These darker herbs, of course, can also be effectively used by people with dark skins.

BODY POWDER LAVENDER FOR MEN AND WOMEN

> 2 oz. Lavender, PO (I use a moulinex coffee
>   grinder to powder herbs)
> 2 oz. fine Montana talc or any other unscented
>   talcum

Mix thoroughly and sift through a fine sieve discarding any large particles. Men particularly like the clean scent of Lavender on their bodies. ½ oz. powdered Lemon peel could also be added and would subtly alter the Lavender scent making a Lavender-Lemon powder that is extremely refreshing.

BODY POWDER FOR MEN

> 2 oz. unscented talcum (if desired)
> 1 oz. powdered Sandalwood (has antiseptic action
>   and is useful in skin diseases)
> 1 oz. powdered Blue Malva or Rose or Vetivert

Mix together thoroughly and then sift through a fine sieve.

BODY POWDER VIOLET

2 oz. unscented talcum

1 oz. powdered Violet flowers (contains vitamins A and C and has a slight antiseptic action when used externally)

1 oz. powdered Orris root (has caused skin allergies in some but the scent is said to relieve headache)

4 drops oil of Violet

2 drops oil of Bitter Almond

Drop the oil of Violet and the oil of Bitter Almond onto the powdered Violet flowers and shake in a closed container. Add the Orris root and shake again. Add the talcum, mix thoroughly, then sift the entire batch through a fine sieve and store in an airtight container or in an old powder box. This powder has a most delightful light scent.

ORANGE-FLOWER POWDER

"Put half a pound of Orange Flowers into a box that contains twelve pounds and a half of powdered Starch; mix them well with the Starch, and ftir the mixture at intervals, to prevent the Flowers from heating. At the expiration of twenty-four hours, remove the old flowers and mix with the Starch the fame quantity of frefh Orange Flowers. Continue acting in this manner for three days together, and if you think the perfume not fufficiently ftrong, add frefh Flowers once or twice more. The box muft be kept clofe fhut as well after as during the operation."

—*The Toilet of Flora,* 1779

This recipe is absolutely delightful but there are few people these days who can get hold of fresh Orange flowers and if they could, they probably would not want to make 13 lbs. of body powder. So, for the same nice powder the following recipe will probably be more than fufficient.

> 1 oz. starch or talcum or cornstarch
> 1 oz. powdered Orange flowers

Mix together and sift through a fine sieve. This Orange-Flower powder is also quite nice and when made with cornstarch is perfect for babies and their eternal diapering.

BLUE POWDER FOR BLUE SKINS
(for our Venerian Friends)

1 part powdered Blue Malva

1 part powdered Bachelor Buttons

1 part powdered Lavender buds

1 part powdered Violet flowers

Mix together and then sift through a fine sieve discarding all large particles. Has a nice natural scent and is useful also as a mild stimulant when the scent is inhaled.

EGGSHELL BODY POWDER

1. 2 dozen powdered eggshells (brown egg for brown skin and white egg for white skin)
2. 1 oz. powdered herbs—Orange peel, Orris root, Cornsilk, Lemon peel, or Licorice root. (Choice depends on the color of your skin and the scent you like.)
3. 8 drops of essential oil—use Violet oil with Orris root, Orange oil with Orange peel, Anise oil with Licorice root, etc.
4. Mix all these things together completely and resift.

Chapter XXII

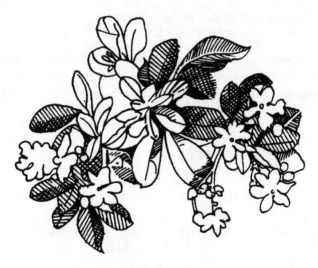

Bath, Body, and Massage Oils

THE ADDITION OF fragrances and fragrant oils to the bath was recorded during early Roman times and Cleopatra has probably done more than anyone to advertise this soothing application of scented oils. Originally, oil was the bath. You would go to a room, and sauna or steam until your pores were relaxed, then a good rub down with a terry towel would remove the released soil. An oil rub down and the removal of the oil with a scraper called a strigil would follow and, finally, a steam bath and a soothing massage with a light oil. The use of the scraper, or a spatula, to remove the outer scaly layer of the skin is still a wonderful addition to the bath. See the Oil Bath in Chapter XXVII.

Apart from the relaxation and hygienic psychological

benefits of a bath, what other extrinsic satisfactions does the introduction of a bath oil provide? Indeed, dermatologists have found the addition of these oils effective in the treatment of dry skin. This annoying problem can result from poor nutrition, metabolic, hormonal, or environmental causes. These natural bath oils will relieve the symptoms of dry, scaling and itching skin; chafed or chapped skin; atopic dermatitis; psoriasis; ichthyosis; soap itch; static itch; winter itch; bath itch; and other types of itches. The application of a thin film of oil to the outer skin provides a barrier to the further loss of moisture. Oil-water compresses can reduce inflammation, itching, irritation, and other skin discomforts.

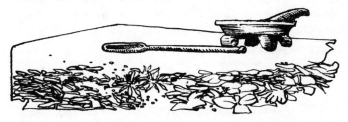

There are two kinds of oils in the bath—floating oils and those that disperse in the water.

The floating oil acts as an emollient to the skin and leaves a pleasant fragrance in the bath, on the body, and in the bathroom. Natural, cold-pressed vegetable oils—such as Olive, peanut, Safflower, wheat germ (vitamin E content), Sesame, Sunflower, Avocado, Soy, fruit kernel oils such as Apricot, Almond, Peach, and some animal oils that have a particular affinity to the human skin such as mink and lanolin—are generally used. (Attention vegetarians: lanolin is *not* the fat from a killed sheep; it is the fat from the wool taken when the sheep is sheared.)

Most commercial bath oils contain mineral oil, and this mineral oil is often sold as "baby oil." In fact, this should not be used either on babies or on your adult skin for it is absorbed through the skin taking the fat soluble vitamins A, D, E, and K along with it. And these vitamins are then excreted through the feces. They also readily dissolve in the mineral oil as it passes through the skin (showing, of course, that the skin does absorb what you put on it), and into the blood stream, thus possibly producing vitamin deficiencies. Indeed, because the body is robbed of these vitamins, mineral oil or any product in which it appears should not be used under any circumstances, though any of the above mentioned vegetable oils may be used in quantity to protect the skin.

I have before me a paper distributed by a major chemical corporation that supplies ingredients to many major cosmetic companies and Formula No. 1, for a Spreading Bath Oil, lists the following ingredients (my comments appear in parentheses):

> 50% by weight: Mineral oil (cheap and readily available)
>
> 35% by weight: Propoxylated medium chain alcohol (reduces the greasy feel of mineral oil and increases the solvent properties of the perfume in the mineral oil)
>
> 10% by weight: Esterified lanolin sterol esters (skin emollient and helps protect the skin from the drying effects of soap. However, most commercial lanolin is synthetic)
>
> 2% by weight: Polypropylene glycol monooleate (makes the oil spread quickly into a thin layer of the bath water)
>
> 3% by weight: Perfume (usually a synthetic, to save money and make money on the consumer)

However, to be perfectly fair, let me mention the one positive fact about mineral oil: It seems to penetrate the skin faster than either lanolin or vegetable oil, and, therefore, the skin is said to lose less moisture with the mineral oil than with lanolin (lanolin 25 per cent reduction in moisture loss and mineral oil 8 per cent). At the same time, mineral oil seems to adhere to the skin better than vegetable oils. But if you use a mixture of vegetable oils and lanolin, the advantages of retaining your vitamins far outweigh the slight advantage of better penetration that the mineral oil might offer.

There are many different types and combinations of oils that one can use in making fine floating bath oils. Here are a few basic recipes that you can enlarge and embroider on depending on what you have at hand or what is available at your health food store. The only vegetable oils I would not recommend are Corn or cottonseed oils because something like 75 per cent of the pesticides and fungicides made in the United States are used solely on the cotton and/or Corn crops and for all of you who wish to limit your intake and accumulation of these poisons, these two should probably be avoided.

FLOATING BATH OILS

BASIC BATH OIL RECIPE (use only cold pressed oils)

½ cup Sesame oil (for vitamins)
½ cup Safflower oil
½ cup Soy oil
½ cup peanut oil
½ cup fruit kernel oil

Add ½ oz. essential oil of anything you like and shake all together thoroughly. Pour some of the oil under the full force of the hot water tap of your tub, jump in and relax.

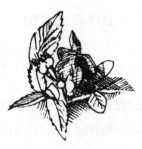

ORIENTAL FLOWER BATH OIL

½ cup Apricot kernel oil
½ cup Sesame seed oil
½ cup Sweet Almond oil

½ cup peanut oil
½ oz. Honeysuckle or
  Jasmine oil

Shake together thoroughly.

CALIFORNIA CITRUS BATH OIL

½ cup Avocado oil
½ cup any fruit kernel
  oil
½ cup Soy oil

½ cup melted
  coconut oil
½ oz. Orange peel oil
½ oz. Lemon peel oil

Shake together thoroughly.

MEDITERRANEAN BATH OIL

½ cup Olive oil
½ cup Sunflower oil
½ cup wheat germ oil
½ cup Safflower oil

½ oz. essential oil of
  Lavender
¼ oz. essential oil of Basil

Shake thoroughly.

THE BULGARIAN ROSE BATH

½ cup Sunflower oil
½ cup Safflower oil
½ cup Sesame oil

½ cup Apricot oil
½ oz. essential oil of Rose
¼ cup essential oil of Violets

Shake thoroughly.

WATER DISPERSIBLE OILS

The *water dispersible oil* is one that immediately dissolves in the water and usually does not leave a ring around the tub.

PERFUMED PROTEIN BATH OIL

Beat 1 egg and ½ cup Safflower oil together until smooth.

Slowly add 1 t. liquid Ivory or other liquid biodegradable detergent and continue to beat. Very slowly add 2 T. alcohol (unscented), or tincture of Benzoin in which ½ t. essential oil has been dissolved to the egg-Ivory-oil mixture until everything is thoroughly incorporated; now, slowly add ¼ cup skim milk and thoroughly mix it all together. You might have an easier time of it if you do this in a blender. Add to your bath.

FRAGRANT DISPERSIBLE BATH OIL

It is very important when using rubbing alcohol to use the unscented kind as the usual alcohol has such a strong smell that it overrides the scent of the essential oil dissolved in it. You could also start with tincture of Benzoin to which you add an essential oil in the proportion of 1:4; that is, ¼ oz. oil to 1 oz. tincture.

1. Melt ¼ cup hydrous lanolin and add slowly, mixing all the while, 1½ cups mixed vegetable oils.
2. Add slowly ½ cup alcohol in which 1 oz. essential oil has been dissolved.
3. Shake all together thoroughly. This substance is milky although the milkiness does not show in the bath and it will disperse immediately in the water.

We rather like this particular bath oil made with essential oil of Lime and ¼ oz. chlorophyll (purchasable in health food stores)—which makes the mixture green and leaves the bath water with a pleasant light green tinge. The bath is slightly slippery and your skin will feel pleasantly smooth, soft, and limily fragrant.

3-LAYER BATH OIL

The only advantage to layered bath oils is that in a pretty, long, thin glass bottle they look very attractive and add interest to the bathroom. They are composed of insoluble ingredients poured or dripped one on top of the other, and when shaken together, blend temporarily. They are poured into the tub and cause the skin to feel smooth.

To make them, just add different ingredients one to the other—you can color water with vegetable food colors, and vegetable oils with oil dyes. One that I like rather well is composed of blue salt water, then oil mixed with wheat germ oil, which is yellow, then tincture of Benzoin (alcohol) mixed with essential oil of Bitter Almond, which is paler yellow.

First, take 2 oz. water and add 4 drops of blue vegetable food coloring and ½ t. salt and shake thoroughly. Pour into a narrow glass bottle. Then mix 1 oz. of vegetable oil with 1 oz. of wheat germ oil fortified with vitamin E, shake thoroughly, and dribble it ever so gently onto the water. Mix 2 oz. tincture of Benzoin with 1 t. Bitter Almond oil, and drool this combination quite slowly over the oil in the bottle.

When I want to use this mix in my bath I shake it up and add anywhere from 2–4 oz. If I don't use all of the layered bath oil, it is put back onto the shelf and sometimes it separates back into three layers, sometimes only into two layers. It hardly ever lasts long enough to make any difference anyway as I would rather make only enough layered bath oil for one bath so that I can keep playing with the colors and scents.

BODY OILS

Body oils are different from bath oils in that they are usually less strongly scented and are put onto the body by massage rather than in the bath. There are two types of body oils: those mixtures that are simply scented with essential oils and which can either smell nice, be used for smoothing wrinkles, and emollients, or if the right mixture of oils is used, be used for aromatherapy; and those mixtures of oils made from herbs for their special properties and which are especially useful in aroma massage.[1]

Take any one oil or mixture of oils you desire and add ¼–1 oz. essential oil to every quart of body oil. I especially like to use mixtures of oils that contain wheat germ fortified with vitamin E—for wrinkles and to improve the texture of the skin.

JEANNE'S SPECIAL BODY AND MASSAGE OIL

1 oz. wheat germ oil fortified with vitamin E + 4 100 i.u. vitamin E capsules pierced with a pin, squeezed, and mixed into the contents. This will provide 400 units of E/oz. of finished oil, a significant amount for dry or wrinkled skin. You could also add vitamin A to provide 15,000 units/oz.; good for blemishes and skin.

1½ oz. Avocado oil, which seems to disappear directly into the skin, for smoothness.

1½ oz. Apricot oil used as a moisturizer and humectant

¼ oz. oil of Carnation for that nice, flowery, spicy scent

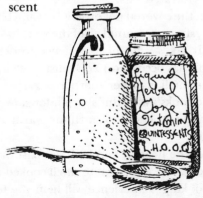

[1]For a more detailed discussion of this fascinating subject, see my future book, *The Herbal Bath & Massage Oil Book*, about how to make massage and body oils and essential oils.

HERBAL MASSAGE OIL

There is another type of body oil, a bit harder to make than the above, but because it is made from herbs, it definitely has more cosmetic and medicinal applications. You can make herbal massage oil by the Hot Method or the Cold Method. The effects that you can get with herbs depend on the herbs that you use.

THE HOT METHOD

1. Put 4 oz. of herbs in a nonmetal pot that will hold about 3 qts. of liquid.
2. Pour over the herbs ½ cup of dry white wine. Cover the pot and let it sit for several hours. The alcohol in the wine starts the extraction of the active substances in the herbs and also keeps the oil from cooking or smelling burned.
3. After a few hours add two quarts of vegetable oil. I consider the best mixture of oils for massage to be cold-pressed Soy, peanut, and Safflower in equal proportions because of their exceptional emolliency and, together, they contain all of the essential nonsaturated fats.
4. Now put the covered pot on low heat and bring it to simmer, simmering until all of the wine has cooked away. (It takes a bit of experience to determine when this has occurred.) You must smell it, and, at first, the smell is rather sharp and grapey. But as the wine cooks away, this sharp odor slowly disappears, and you begin to smell the warm scents of the herbs.
5. Turn off the heat. If you let it get past this warm herb scent, you will begin to smell cooked oil. Too much cooking! Experience will help you to determine the difference between a grapey, an herby, and a burny oil smell.

6. Let the oil cool in the pot and then strain through cheesecloth or muslin into a half-gallon container.
7. Let the oil settle—in about a week there may be a slight separation at the bottom of the container.
8. Decant the clear oil into another clean container and discard the residue. (This residue contains the rest of the wine that wasn't cooked off and usually some of the natural plant dyes.)
9. Now, if you wish, add about ½–1 oz. essential oil to the clear massage oil to scent it.

There are several pieces of equipment which come in handy if you make a lot of massage oil: A metal funnel that has a small screen in it is useful when you are straining out herbs; there is a metal ball with holes all the way round —which can be bought in specialty stores for kitchen goodies and is commonly used for cooking rice—that is very nice for either putting bath herbs into and dropping into the tub, or for putting massage oil herbs into, then closing the ball and adding the wine, the oil, and cooking. It makes straining that much easier. Certainly, use wooden spoons for scraping or stirring as the less metal that comes into contact with the herbs the better.

Now what herbs should you use? The variety and mixture is infinite depending on the results you wish to obtain. See *Herbs & Things* for the medicinal use of herbs and this book, Chapter I, for the cosmetic uses.

GREEN OIL

1 oz. Alfalfa-CS
2 oz. Parsley-CS
1 oz. Comfrey leaf-CS

Follow the recipe for the Hot Method of making massage oil. Scent with oil of sage or patchouli or sandalwood.

MASSAGE OIL FOR SUPPLE LIMBS

2 oz. Henna herb-CS
1 oz. Comfrey root-CS
1 oz. Sage-CS

Follow the recipe for the Hot Method of making massage oil. Scent with oil of Sage.

MASSAGE OIL FOR OVER-FLAGGING BREASTS

1 oz. Lady's mantle-CS   1 oz. Woodruff-CS
1 oz. Quince seed   1 oz. Comfrey leaf-CS
   —mashed in a mortar
   and pestle

Follow the recipe for either the Hot Method or Cold Method of making massage oil. Scent this massage oil with the Vanilla oil which you can purchase from Indiana Botanic (Chapter VI). The Vanilla oil will bead up in this massage mixture, but it is the best smelling and best tasting, so just shake your oil thoroughly each time before using. Another good alternative would be to scent the oil with pure essential oil of Ylang-ylang—however, most stores sell only the synthetic (it doesn't matter that they claim to have the pure, they really only have synthetic). (See also Chapter XVIII.)

This mixture is considered to be quite erotic and sensual by many men; it could be that Vanilla reminds them of home, mother, and those comforting milky smells of childhood.

CELLULITE MASSAGE OIL

2 oz. Strawberry leaves-CS
1 oz. Sage
1 oz. Jaborandi
¼ oz. Sage essential oil
or

Witch Hazel leaves-CS
Marigold
Camomile
Lemon essential oil
or
1 oz. Linden
1 oz. Pennyroyal
1 oz. Orange leaves
¼ oz. Mint oil

Follow the recipe for the Hot Method of making massage oil and also read Chapter XVII for further information about these dread bulges.

THE COLD METHOD OF MAKING MASSAGE OILS

Basically the cold method means made with no heat. It is used for those plants, herbs, and flowers having delicate scents which would be unfavorably altered by the heat of cooking. The end result is a massage oil less strongly, albeit more naturally, colored by the natural herbs—and more naturally scented. Cold pressed oils retain their natural vitamins and minerals while solvent, extracted oils go through many processes that destroy vitamins and minerals before they are available for use. I used to think that it was ridiculous to use cold pressed oils in the Hot Method because the heat destroyed their vitamins and minerals; because it is generally more expensive to use them it seemed silly to spend the extra money for the cold pressed oils just to destroy their cold-pressedness by heat. However, Rodale's *Prevention Magazine* says there is *no* information that temperatures up to 475° destroy vitamins, minerals, or enzymes. So, by all means use cold pressed oils in all recipes for massage or body oils.

THE COLD METHOD

1. Take about 4 oz. of herbs, fresh or dried, and put them into a nonmetal pot or brown glass bottle that will hold about 3 qts. of liquid
2. Pour over the herbs about ½ cup of dry white wine. Cover the pot or bottle and let it sit for a couple of hours. The alcohol in the wine starts the extraction of the active substances in the herbs.
3. After a few hours add 2 qts. of slightly heated—not hot, just warm—vegetable oil. Cover the pot again and let it sit for 1 day to 1 week in the hot sun.
4. When the oil has taken on the aroma of the herbs, strain it through cheesecloth into a clean glass container.
5. After a period of time the oil will separate from the wine, and then, you decant the clear oil off the top. Now add ¼–1 oz. essential oil, as you wish.

REJUVENATING MASSAGE OIL

1 oz. Ginseng-PO

1 oz. Red Rose buds or petals-CS

1 oz. Jamaica flowers-CS

1 oz. Comfrey root-CS or PO

Scent with *pure* essential oil of Rose. Follow the recipe for the Cold Method.

SUMMER EROTIC MASSAGE OIL

1 oz. fresh Honeysuckle flowers

1 oz. fresh Honeysuckle leaves

1 oz. fresh Jasmine flowers (or dry)

1 oz. sweet Brier leaves

(also called Eglantine Rose), or if unavailable, use Red Rose buds or petals

¼–1 oz. *pure* oil of Honeysuckle or Jasmine, whichever is available

Follow the recipe for the Cold Method.

Again, this brings to mind a small brochure that I have from a "Body Shop" here in San Francisco that caters to the common individual's ignorance about essential oils. As you know, "Essential Oils" are defined as the "essence or the essential nature of something, its intrinsic character, the part that is unchangeable and permanent, the very root and heart and being of it. The essential oil of a plant or flower possesses the fragrance virtues of the plant or flower in concentrated form. An essential oil is a volatile oil as distinguished from a fixed oil in that it evaporates with comparative ease, especially in the presence of steam. . . ." (*Perfume Album*, by Jill Jessee). This company, on the one hand, puts down the larger cosmetic companies as being dishonest and selling cheap ingredients at a grossly inflated price, but, on the other hand, sells its own essential oils as "organic" and mentions that their own oils derive their scent from real plants or flowers. Half their essential oils have never even been close to a plant or flower, but, instead, derive their scent purely in the chemist's laboratory. Whoever heard of musk oil coming from a flower? But then, maybe, they actually mean Ambrette oil, in which case they should say Ambrette, and not musk. And pure Jasmine and Rose oil are so wonderfully expensive that they could not possibly be sold at $1.00/¼ oz. So be not deceived, most flower and essential oils are synthetic. The following list of oils is generally in this synthetic category:

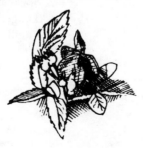

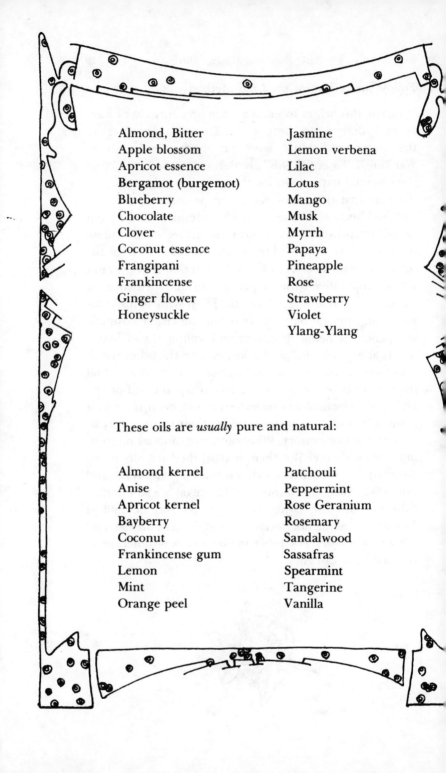

Almond, Bitter	Jasmine
Apple blossom	Lemon verbena
Apricot essence	Lilac
Bergamot (burgemot)	Lotus
Blueberry	Mango
Chocolate	Musk
Clover	Myrrh
Coconut essence	Papaya
Frangipani	Pineapple
Frankincense	Rose
Ginger flower	Strawberry
Honeysuckle	Violet
	Ylang-Ylang

These oils are *usually* pure and natural:

Almond kernel	Patchouli
Anise	Peppermint
Apricot kernel	Rose Geranium
Bayberry	Rosemary
Coconut	Sandalwood
Frankincense gum	Sassafras
Lemon	Spearmint
Mint	Tangerine
Orange peel	Vanilla

PYRAMID MASSAGE OIL

2 oz. Camomile flowers (fresh if possible)
1 oz. Marigold flowers
1 oz. Lemon peel (if you use the fresh, use both
the white of the peel for the bioflavenoids
and the peel itself for scent and vitamin C)
¼ oz. oil of Lemon, if desired

Follow the recipe for the Cold Method. This oil smooths the skin, relaxes the muscles, and its scent is thought to relax the mind as well. I also call this oil Egyptian Massage Oil.

The average Lemon with the peel contains 77 milligrams of ascorbic acid per 100 grams of edible portion, while the Lemon, peeled, contains only 53 milligrams of ascorbic acid per 100 grams of edible portion. There is more vitamin C in the peel than in the rest of the Lemon and the same is true of the Orange. Orange peel contains 136 mg. of ascorbic acid, the Orange with the peel contains 71 mg., and Orange juice contains only 50 mg. (from *Compositions and Facts about Foods*, by Ford Heritage). Herbs contain even more vitamin C than citrus. Strawberry leaves 229 mg.; Violet leaves 210 mg.; catnip 83 mg.; and Nettle 76 mg.

SODOM-ME OIL (Hot or Cold Method)

1 oz. Comfrey root, for healing and emolliency
1 oz. Mugwort, for relaxing the muscles, soothing
them, and maybe to open the third eye
1 oz. Quince seed, for astringency to give firm-
ness to the flesh
1 oz. Thyme, for its antiseptic qualities
¼ oz. fragrance of chocolate, if desired

Substitute 1 cup of melted Cocoa butter (used for its exceptional emolliency) for 1 cup of the vegetable oil in the Cold Method when making the massage oil.

There are many, many more massage oils you can make by either the hot or the cold method. Keep in mind that the cold method is most useful for delicate plants to conserve their more subtle, easily destroyed scents, while the hot method probably extracts more of the plant's cosmetic elements. Decide what type of oil you want to make and the purpose you wish for it, then use Chapter I for the names of those plants which will accomplish your purpose. There are a few companies that make massage oils with herbs, and their addresses are in Chapter VI.

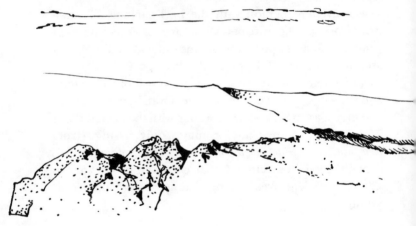

TABLE OF OILS

The following oils are nondrying and especially useful for dry skin. Nondrying oils contain mostly saturated and oleic acid glycerides with very little to no linoleic or linolenic acids. Upon exposure to air they remain liquid for long periods of time and have a low iodine number (less than 100). Nondrying oils are usually extracted from tropical plants: Almond, Castor, Cocoa butter, Olive, Palm, peanut, and Rape are all nondrying.

Semidrying oils do not have much linolenic acid but have quite a bit of linoleic acid and more saturated acids; they dry slowly upon exposure to air and at higher temperatures and have an iodine number of 100–130. These oils are more suitable for normal to oily skins: corn, cottonseed, Croton, Sesame, and Sunflower are all types of semidrying oils.

Drying oils are very high in the unsaturated glycerides, most especially linoleic and linolenic acid. They are quite low in oleic acid, they dry slowly in the air to form a film, and have a high iodine number (over 130). Usually these oils come from plants that make their home in temperate climates. Drying oils are more suitable for oily skins but are generally best used mixed with other oils: linseed, Hempseed, Soybean, Tung, and most nut oils are drying.

Chapter XXIII

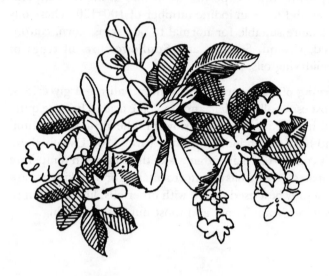

Aromatherapy – Colognes and Perfumes

Aromatherapy is the use of aromatic substances and volatile oils by inhalation or direct absorption through pressure point massage to treat mental and physical difficulties. One aim of cosmetic Aroma-massage is to slow down the aging process of the skin through cellular regeneration. At Essential in Beverly Hills I have undergone the treatment and loved every second of the application of the oils. Delightful! When the oils penetrate the skin they act as regulators, to balance and to counteract the negative effects of a poor physical and mental environment.

Essential oils are used as perfumes but they also have other purposes: Vanilla, to revive warm, loving memories of mother; a combination of Apricot, wheat germ, Sandalwood, Lavender, and Lemon, to treat oily skin and acneic conditions; a combination of Peppermint, Menthol, and Bay by inhalant therapy and external massage is helpful for congested tissues whether on the outside of the body or from a cold; Dalmatian Sage for intoxication and giddiness; Thymol to bring forth memories of early medical traumas; Heliotrope, for garden memories and increasing sexual emotions; Benzoin and Canella for nervous fatigue; Rose and Rosemary to increase energy; Anise and Fennel to open up the facial pores; Melissa to calm a racing heart; Birch to treat skin disease; Borage to strengthen the adrenals; Camomile for the skin and as a nerve sedative; Carnation to increase sexual desires (I have used it while pregnant to massage my abdomen and have found that it eases the pain of contractions); Orange, Camomile, Willow, or Rose to hydrate the skin; Marigold to cheer the heart or for grief; Marjoram for those who sigh too much; Melilot helps melancholy and for people who have lost their senses; Motherwort oil massage for cramps and to ward off evil spirits; Pansy for babies; Rose for memory and hay fever; Rosemary for forgetfulness; Wild Strawberry used as pressure point massage is said to affect the points that control the lymphatic glands of the gut; Violet for sleep and headaches; Woodruff for the bile ducts.

This is a subject which has been studied by only a few persons, including Knutt Larrson, a Swedish doctor, of Goteborg University. He has proven that there is an interdependence between sexuality and odor and that there is a connection between how one perceives odor and impotence—in other words, the genital nerves and the olfactory nerves are in some way related.

André Virel is a French psychoanalyst who worked with persons who were unable to remember long-buried pain and traumas. By wafting cotton balls scented with certain essential oils under the nose of his patients, he brought forth these hidden memories. He is said to have used

Vanillin, which seems to be related to the scent of mother's milk or at least mother's cooking, to help his patients remember scenes of earliest childhood. In my classes at the University of California Extension in San Francisco about 60 per cent of the students associate Vanilla-scented blotters with cooking and baking. These memories are invariably pleasant.

A. H. Conney and J. J. Burns, in an article entitled "Metabolic Interactions Among Environmental Chemicals and Drugs," found that chemicals in man's environment such as volatile oils, alter the action of drugs by stimulating microsomal enzyme activity in animals.

Marguerite Maury, a French biologist, claims to have discovered the power of a number of odors to stimulate or balance various bodily functions. She used Lavender to fight muscular fatigue and—when incorporated into a pillow—to help promote sound sleep.

You can apply aromatherapy at home with a few basic tools. First, you must obtain the very best high quality *pure* essential oils. This is, at times, most difficult. Kiehl Pharmacy in New York has some wonderful essential oils. Also Wide World Herbs in Canada and P. Robertet, Co. of Paris, London, and New York have absolutely exquisite odors, but I do not know if they have retail outlets. In Chapter XXII of this book is a list of oils that when bought from the usual pharmacy, herb store, "body" shop, or chemist shop are invariably synthetic. The proprietors of these stores will usually tell you that the oils are pure, pure synthetic, yes, but not pure natural oils. Please do not use these synthetic oils for aromatherapy.

EXTENDING PURE OIL

After you have obtained your pure oil you can dilute it so that it will last longer. Put about ⅛–¼ oz. oil into a 1 oz. bottle. Fill the bottle with Apricot kernel or Sweet Almond

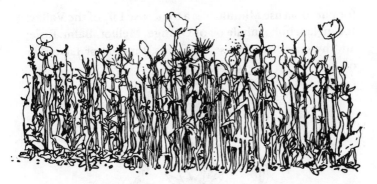

oil as a carrier oil, seal, and put the bottle away in a cool dark place to age, so that the carrier oil will take on the scent of the essential oil.

Now you can use the oil in pressure point massage or simply inhale it to get the effects you want. There are a few places that practice and/or know about aroma massage; besides the Aroma Salons in London and Paris there is Essential in Beverly Hills, Renaissance in the Bahamas, and probably others that I am unaware of.

VAPOUR ROOM

The hot scented air of vapour rooms at noted spas around the world is thought to have a salutary effect on one's metabolism and circulation. They can soften and improve the texture of the skin and induce a pleasant frame of mind. You can have a vapour room at home—very easily—by converting your bathroom with the simple addition of a hot plate or electric skillet. Run a hot bath; somewhere away from the tub plug in an electric skillet. Turn the skillet low and add your herbs or flowers. Add an oil such as Safflower or coconut. Heat the oil and let the herbs simmer. Add a few drops of essential oil. Sit in your herbal bath and inhale the cleansing aromas. If you are subject to bad dreams, inhale the scent of Anise, Cloves, Ginseng, or Rosemary. To exhilarate the brain, use Dill;

for paranoia use Mimulus; as a tonic, use Lily of the Valley; for melancholy, inhale oil of Orange, Melilot, Balm, Rose; and hysterics should use Narcissus, Linden, or Lavender oil.

COLOGNES AND PERFUMES

You can also make essential oils at home—maybe not with the quality of the essential oils of Grasse but perfectly acceptable for home use. With these oils you can then go on and make colognes and perfumes.

ENFLEURAGE

Simply apply a layer of pure lard or rendered fat to a glass frame or enamel pan. Many thick-petaled flowers such as Jasmine, Tuberose, and Honeysuckle produce their oils long after they have been picked. So place one layer of freshly picked flowers on the fat and leave them for 24–36 hours. After this, remove the flowers and put new ones on the frame. Repeat until your fat has the scent you desire—about 1 week should do it. At the end of this time remove the last of the flowers and scrape the fat into a container. Keep the frames in a warm, but dry place. Add a few drops of compound tincture of benzoin to the fat as a preservative if you like, but it often alters the scent of the pure flower oils.

COLOGNE

You can use the fat as above or you can digest the scented

fat in quadruple its *weight* of pure alcohol (about 2½ to 3 cups alcohol to 6 oz. of oil). Rubbing alcohol will not do. The pure alcohol absorbs the essential oil from the fat in time. After several months skim the fat and then dilute the scented alcohol with water to make cologne.

TUBEROSE WINE

I use this method when my Tuberose comes into bloom in the spring. Each of the bulbs produces a flower stalk that in turn produces flowers daily for about 1–2 weeks. On each stalk 1–3 flowers open per day. Since I have only about 3 dozen bulbs, I use my flowers mainly to make flower champagne (see the Wine Method) and with what's left —which is very little—I make oil of Tuberose using a tiny glass frame about 6 inches x 6 inches. Tuberose has to be picked just prior to opening in order to yield the most fragrant oil. It takes 3600 kilos of flowers to make 1 kilo of Tuberose absolute.

THE MAYONNAISE METHOD

You can make scented oils by the methods suggested in Chapter XXII. Or fill a large mayonnaise jar with flowers and add warm Olive oil to just cover the flowers. If it is a hot day, the oil will take on the scent of the flowers within 24 hours, if not it may take 36 hours. Strain out the flowers, add a bit of compound tincture of Benzoin to the oil, and keep in a cool, dry place until needed. This type of oil can be used as a perfume oil, scented body oil, or massage oil. Honeysuckles take very well to this method.

SOLVENT EXTRACTION WITH ETHYL ALCOHOL

You will need either high-proof vodka or pure ethyl alcohol. Fill a jar with crushed dried herbs or spices. Add alcohol to just cover the herb. Tighten down the lid of the jar, *shake thoroughly every day,* and steep from 1–4 weeks or longer depending on the botanical. If the scent is still not strong enough, strain out the material, and add more. Don't try to smell the tincture of alcohol directly—dip a piece of pure white blotting paper into it, wave it about until the alcohol has evaporated off and then smell. When it smells right use it directly or mix with other tinctures to develop a perfume. You can also strain this substance through coffee filter papers to obtain a clear tincture.

THE BACH WAY

Another method of extracting oils from flowers is to simply float the flowers on pure spring water in the sun and collect on cotton-tipped sticks the oil that floats to the top. See *Herbs & Things,* p. 169.

HOW TO GATHER AND CLARIFY MAY-DEW

When there hath fallen no raine the night before, then with a cleane and large sponge, the next morning, you may gather the same from sweet herbs, grasse or corne: straine your dew, and expose it to the Sun in glasses covered with papers or parchment prickt full of holes; strain it often, continuing it in the Sun, & in a hot place, till the same grow white and cleare, which will require the best part of the Summer.

Some comment May-Dew, gathered from Fennell and Celandine, to be most excellent for sore eyes; and some commend the same (prepared as before) above Rosewater for preserving of fruits, flowers, &c.

—*Delightes for Ladies*

TO MAKE ESSENCE OF CINNAMON

Take a half a pound of Cinnamon, reduce it in a mortar to an impalpable powder, put it into a very long-necked matrafs, pour on it as much highly rectified Spirit of Wine as will cover the powder, about an inch. Stop the matrafs with a found cork coated with bees-wax, and expose it to the sun for a whole month, observing to shake it well twice a day. At the expiration of the month, uncork the matrafs, using the utmost precaution not to disturb the sediment; and gently pour off the Tincture into a clean vial.

—*The Toilet of Flora,* 1779

Of course, the easiest method of making perfume is to mix together various essential oils to suit your sense of smell. To make colognes, dissolve the essential oils in 4 times their amount of alcohol. Let it digest in the alcohol for some time, add 5 times that amount of pure spring water and you will have a cologne.

DESIRÉE'S FAVORITE PERFUME

Desirée uses her homemade Honeysuckle oil made by the Mayonnaise Method and mixes equal amounts with Violet oil, oil of Spanish Jasmine, and oil of Carnation. The latter three she purchases from Kiehl's in New York. She mixes only ⅛ oz. at a time, dissolves this in 1 oz. of Apricot oil, lets it stand for a month in a cool dark place, and then uses it at the pulse points—wrists, breasts, inner arms, and the soft skin between the thighs. It is very effective.

THE WINE METHOD

I like to use white wine—usually a German variety will work better than a French—to soak herbs in. We drink this wine, cook with it, or use it as a last rinse for clothing. The clothing takes on the scent of the botanical obviating the need for colognes. Rose, Apple, Peppermint, or Geranium wine is delightful by this method, as is Tuberose, Carnation, and Woodruff wine.

Like the Romans, I like to put different scents on different parts of my body. This way, when I need a mood change I just sniff the proper place; Mimosa on the left arm reminds me of dirt roads in the summer along which are golden yellow trees; Absolute Oeillet inside the left elbow is for warmth and comfort; Rose Turque on the right arm to ease tension, and Ginger Africa for stimulation.

TO UNSTICK PERFUME BOTTLES

If the stopper is stuck, cover with a film of glycerin and jiggle the stopper. Continue applying glycerin every hour or so until it is unstuck.

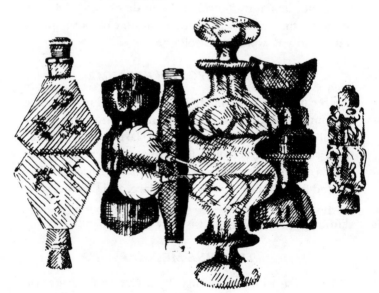

Chapter XXIV

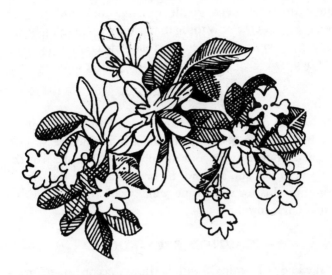

The Hands, Feet, Fingernails, Elbows, Knees, Chest, and Breasts

THE CHEST area often sadly neglected and which often collects lumps of fat needs attention and love too.

FOR WRINKLES THAT OCCUR BELOW THE HOLLOW OF THE THROAT AND ABOVE THE BREASTS

Take 2 oz. White Lily root juice and mix with an equal amount of honey. Add 1 oz. of melted yellow beeswax and 1 oz. of melted lanolin. Mix together completely, beat until cold, and pot up for use. Apply every night and remove every morning. This salve can be used on any wrinkles that occur on the face or body.

Breasts need exercise to strengthen the muscles that hold them up; they need gentle massage and moisturizers. Some say that the only thing that can alter a sagging breast is surgery while others feel the following creams regularly applied will keep a bosom firm and young looking.

BEAUTIFUL BREAST OIL

Buy a cake of Cocoa butter and melt a little every night in the hands; massage some into and around the breast starting at the outside with your thumbs on the nipples; roll the fingers under and around the breasts and up the center; continue this for some time. Finally rub them dry with a small linen towel.

BEAUTIFUL BREAST OIL #2

Make Lady's Mantle Oil with Safflower according to directions in Chapter XXII. To 3 oz. of this oil, add 1 oz. melted lanolin, 1 oz. wheat germ oil and scent with oil of Rose. Massage your breasts as above.

BEAUTIFUL BREAST OIL #3

Massage your breasts as indicated with wheat germ oil, or castor oil scented with Vanilla, Rose, or Ylang-Ylang. All these things have time honoured reputations as restorers of overflagging breasts.

HANDS AND FINGERNAILS

My husband, who is used to my herbal experiments, was somewhat nonplussed when on an evening in July in 1973 he came down from his studio to go to bed and found me only with a pair of gloves on, the left hand encased in cotton to the wrist and the right in soft kid to the elbow. Inside the pair of gloves was a pair of hands lathered in a mixture of:

SOFT HANDS PASTE FOR DETERGENT OR ROUGH HANDS

> 2 heaping T. Almond meal or Oatmeal
> 1 T. honey
> 1 egg yolk beaten frothy yellow

Mix these ingredients all together.

In the morning my hands were soft, white, and smooth. This paste or a variation, has been used to soften and whiten sore or rough hands for hundreds of years. The variations include additions of Cornmeal, borax, vinegar, or milk. A friend of mine who has had raw, detergent hands for years and who has spent pots of money on dermatologists and medications swears by the efficacy of this paste. She used it every night for a month, while, in the meantime, she confined dishwashing to once a day instead of three times, and in the space of 2 weeks her hands were healed, in 3 weeks soft and in 4 beautiful. The choice of gloves is also very important—although the cottom is considerably less expensive than the kid; it leaks the paste through its pores and onto the bed. Also, the paste dries out somewhat. Kid gloves keep the paste inside and moist and have a synergistic effect on the hands. I prefer kid gloves. As a matter of fact, it would be nice to have a pair of kid socks also, to soften the toes and feet.

ANOTHER PASTE FOR THE HANDS AND FEET

Beat some Almonds in a mortar with a pestle and add some Apple cider vinegar slowly; add 2 t. powdered Benzoin, 2 oz. honey, 2 hard-boiled egg yolks, and beat it all together into a paste. Massage this paste into the hands and take a bath or wear it with kid gloves to bed.

ANOTHER PASTE #3

Mix Almond meal with milk and white bread crumbs until thoroughly incorporated. Add more milk and simmer in a double boiler until it has formed a paste—all the while stirring constantly. Apply as above.

ANOTHER PASTE #4

Mix together equal quantities of Almond meal, Orris root, powdered Sandalwood, Calamus. Add enough Rosewater to moisten the whole; add wheat bread crumbs and work into a paste with mucilage of Tragacanth or Quince that has been made with Rosewater. Apply as above.

CALLOUSED HANDS, BRITTLE NAILS OR CALLOUSED FEET

All these afflictions will benefit from a hot Olive oil soak with added Sage or Red Clover. This also is an excellent moisturizer for the hands, face, or around the eyes.

SIMPLE CHAPPED HANDS OR FEET CURE

Mix Almond oil equally with crystallized honey and apply thickly to the hands or feet. Put on a pair of kid gloves or soft leather socks. Wear the night through. In the morning give your appendages a hot soak in decoction of Pine needles or Burdock. Pat dry.

CHAPPED HANDS

Wheat oil is used for chapped hands, as well as softened lanolin, Almond oil, or Sesame oil.

HANDWATER TO SOFTEN

Take a handful of Lavender, some Cloves, and some Orris root and drop them into some spring water. Bring to a boil, turn off the heat and infuse until cold and strain. Add 1–4 drops of tincture of Benzoin to every ounce of the strained water. Shake together—it will turn milky. Use this solution as a last rinse whenever you wash your hands. You may also use the infusion in your fingerbowls at the table.

TO SOFTEN AND TO REMOVE STAINS FROM THE HANDS

Use the juice of the Sorrel or the Lemon to remove stains and objectionable aromas from the hands. Also, rub the underside of a Lemon, Grapefruit, or Lime peel or a piece of raw Potato on the stain to bleach it out.

BROWN SPOTS

Brown spots on the hands can be considerably lightened by the application of vitamin E and wheat germ oil.

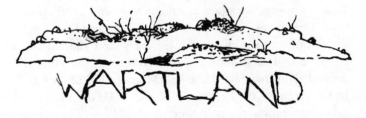

TO CURE WARTS ON THE HANDS

Rub the warts daily with juice of Campanula, Blue Bell flowers, Ivy, inner rind of Lemon steeped in vinegar, Red Onion, juice of the Mercury. In each case after rubbing, apply a bandage (soaked in the juice) for 24 hours and then repeat the process until the wart softens and eventually disappears.

#15. TO TAKE CHILBLANES
OUT OF THE HANDS OR FEET

Boil half a peck of Oats in a quart of water, till they wex dry: then having first anointed your hands with some good Pomatum and well chafed them, hold them within the Oats as hot as you may well suffer them, covering the bowl wherein you put your hands, with a double cloth, to keep in the steam of the Oats. Do this three or four times, and you shall find the effect. The same Oats will serve to be sodden with fresh water three or four times.

—*Delightes for Ladies*

THE NAILS

Fingernails and toenails are there to guard the fingers and toes. The are composed of protein called keratin; growth occurs only at the point where the nail enters the fingers—or toes—in a place called the matrix. Take care of your nails regularly on a weekly basis. Start by soaking your toes and fingers in soap and water—a bath will do it. Take an orange stick (a manicuring tool) and gently push back the cuticles, clean the nails with a natural bristle nail brush and soap and water. Dry them and file with an emery board in a gentle curve. Never cut the cuticles, instead daily massage in a cuticle cream or any of the lanolin creams in Chapters VIII and XIII. Circulation is very important to the nails, and they will benefit by a good supply of blood. So be sure to get your exercise every day. Bumps, ridges, and marks on the nails are a result of injury and do not appear until sometime after the injury has occurred. Illnesses also can result in reduced nail growth. Pregnancy as well as typing or piano playing increases nail growth as well as do buffing or massaging the fingers.

Horizontal ridges occur during menstrual periods and vertical ridges indicate anemia, age, or dryness. Pale color indicates anemia, blue means insufficient oxygen or inefficient circulation. Toxicity to certain drugs shows up in discolored nails. Thin nails, slow-growing nails, or hair, may indicate deficiencies of vitamins, minerals, or protein. Protein deficiency may show up as a flat tapered cuticle or as hangnails. Frequent hangnails can also indicate a lack of folic acid or vitamin C. A high rounded nail may signal respiratory inflammation or too much anticoagulant.

NAIL CARE DO'S AND DON'TS
(This includes the toenails, too)

1. Do push the cuticles back with a soft cloth every time you wash your hands.
     Don't cut cuticles with a scissors.
2. Do wash your nails daily with a natural bristle brush and clean with an orange stick.
     Don't use metal nail files either to clean under your nails or to push back the cuticles.
3. Do file your nails only with an emery board.
     Don't file with a metal file.
4. Do massage with a moisturizing herbal cream, or any cream, into your hands and nails daily, and after every chore, to obtain beautiful, soft, smooth hands.
5. Do eat a balanced, nutritional, natural diet, rest and exercise well for beautiful hands and an attractive body.

GARDENING HINT

For work in the garden, coat your hands with a good cream, and stab your fingernails into a bar of soap or a jar of cream, and then put on a pair of gloves; when you are finished working, your hands and nails will be that much easier to clean.

A LINIMENT TO PROMOTE THE GROWTH AND REGENERATION OF THE NAILS

Apply a mixture of 1 t. of Manna, Aloes[1], and Frankincense and 6 t. of beeswax. Melt the wax, mix this all together and apply around the edges of the fingernails.

ROSE PASTE FINGERNAIL MAKE-UP

Soak ½ oz. powdered Alkanet in 4 oz. vegetable oil for 2 weeks. Strain or not. Melt about ¼ oz. beeswax, add the herbed oil and heat until well incorporated. Add a few drops Otto of Rose (optional). Pot up for use. Apply the paste directly to the nails, rub in, and leave it on for a while. Buff with a nail buffer.

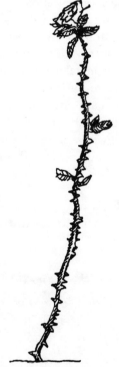

[1]Since this is an adaption of an old formula, Aloes could mean Senna.

HENNA PASTE FINGERNAIL MAKE-UP

Make a paste of Henna and water and with a small brush, paint it on your nails. Leave the paste on for 10 minutes to an hour. Wash off and buff. This will leave a nice, warm color on your nails that will not wash off but only wear off gradually. Reapply at any time.

KNEES

Knees can be beautified with exercise and cream. Combine equal amounts of ripe Avocado and salt. Mash together and rub firmly—with great vigor—into the knees, or, for that matter, any other part of your body that needs softening and stimulation. Then take a nice herb bath.

FEET

Feet like care and attention and feel very badly when they are neglected. They need massage and nail care and nice natural shoes, such as Earth Shoes or Space Shoes, to walk in. (Earth Shoes by Kalsø of Copenhagen, 117 East 17th Street, New York; Murray Space Shoes, 616 Fairfield Avenue, Bridgeport, Connecticut) Besides good shoes for walking, one of the nicest and most invigorating things in the world is to have a professional or a loved one give you a generous foot massage.

FOOT BATHS

Foot baths made up of the following herbs are extremely efficacious as restoratives for poor, tired feet: Alder, Agrimony, Comfrey, Lavender, Pine needles, Yarrow, Red Clover, Sage, Burdock, Houseleek, Mustard seed (circulation), Goats Rue, Rosemary, Witch Hazel, Elderberries, Hayflowers (terrific), Fern, Mugwort, or Melilot. These herbs are effective for all sorts of foot problems excluding ingrown toenails, corns, blisters, and itchy or sweaty feet. For feet that tire out too quickly and don't get you where you want to go, try placing sprigs of Mugwort in your shoes or a sprinkle of Cayenne as a stimulant.

OIL RUBS

Oil rubs made of Safflower oil, wheat germ oil, or Avocado oil and Marigold, Mugwort, Pine needles, Alder, or Comfrey are especially good.

MASSAGE

Massage your feet with Rosemary oil, wetted salt, baking soda, or an Avocado pit, and then soak them in one of the above mentioned foot baths. Very, very invigorating.

FEEL GOOD FEET

Feet will feel better if you occasionally massage them, wear socks filled with dried peas or beans for a few minutes a day to decrease static electricity and for exercise, change your shoes and the height of your heels frequently, wear loose socks and hose, elevate your feet whenever you can, rub them briskly in the shower with a loofah or friction brush, use contrast baths for cramps—Comfrey root in the hot and Witch Hazel in the cold—pick up marbles with your toes, practice moving each toe independently of the others in clockwise circles and use pressure point massage to release the hard little knots that collect on the feet.

A SOOTHING FOOT BATH

Boil in spring water, 1 lb. of Bran, 1 oz. Marshmallow root, and 3 handfuls of Marshmallow or Blue Malva leaves.

AN AROMATIC FOOT BATH

Mix together 1 oz. of each of Pennyroyal, Sage, Rosemary, Angelica, and Juniper berries. Make a decoction and pour into a shallow tub. Put your feet into the tub, resting on the herbs and cover it all up with a thick terry towel to keep the steam in. Relax and when the water is cool, pat your feet

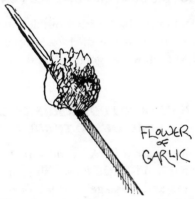

FLOWER of GARLIC

dry, put on slippers and socks, or go to bed. This is very, very nice for sore, tired feet.

CORN REMEDY

This is an old, corn remedy from an older herbal. Roast an Onion or a Garlic clove and apply it hot to the corn; bind with a soft bandage. The corn will loosen and can be removed in 2 or 3 days. Apply hot herb fomentations every other night and then renew the Garlic or Onion applications.

. . . AND AVOCADO FOOT SOFTENER

Beulah Roth has written an absolutely fantastic book just on the wonders of the Avocado for skin care, *The Fresh Avocado Beauty Book.* This recipe is from her book:

Mash the pulp of a ripe Avocado to a thick purée. To this add the juice of half a Lemon and a tablespoon of castor oil. Blend well and rub into the toes, soles, heels, or any other part of the foot which needs softening. Cover with white socks and leave on overnight. Wash thoroughly in the morning with a nail brush, hot water, and soap to loosen all the dead skin.

COCOA BUTTER FOOT SOFTENER

Rub your feet in the bath with a pumice stone. Dry them and apply a cream made of 1 oz. Cocoa butter, 1 oz. Marshmallow root, wheat germ oil, and 1 oz. yellow beeswax.

AVOCADO HAND AND FOOT SCRUB TO CARRY AWAY CALLOUSED TISSUE

In your hands, mash 1 T. Avocado with 1 or 2 T. Cornmeal. Rub your hands together, squish your fingers about, interlock them and massage each joint—one at a time—with a bit of this meal. Very cleansing and softening.

COMFREY ROOT CAMPHOR BALL FOR CHAPPED PLACES

1 oz. yellow beeswax	1 t. sage honey
4 T. Comfrey or sage oil[1]	1 oz. Camphor, PO

Melt the wax and beat in the oil, honey, and camphor until well blended. Beat until cold. Rub on chapped hands, legs, or lips whenever necessary. This is also good for skiers' sunburned or cracked lips.

AVOCADO ELBOW, HEEL, AND KNEE ABRASIVE

If you have hard horny tissue on any of these places, take a piece of Avocado peel and scrape away the meat. The inner part of the peel contains a potent cosmetic oil. The

[1]Make comfrey oil by simmering 1 oz. Comfrey root in 2 cups vegetable oil until the herb is crisp. Cool, strain and use.

peel will feel slightly abrasive; rub this on your elbows, knees or heels, wherever there is any horny tissue. First it will feel oily and leave your skin green, then as you rub it will feel more abrasive. The dead skin seems to dissolve and your elbows will feel satiny smooth. Rub any excess oil into the skin as a moisturizer.

LEMON TO BLEACH THE ELBOWS AND KNEES

Lemons soften and bleach the skin and a Lemon rub on the feet will help to soften a callous. While giving a manicure cut a Lemon in half and stick your elbows in the Lemon. When you have finished your manicure, the elbows will be soft and delicate.

GLYCERIN AND ROSEWATER OR
GLYCERIN AND ORANGEFLOWER WATER
FOR HANDS, FEET, KNEES, OR ELBOWS

Mix equal quantities of glycerin and Rosewater and slather generously on the hands, legs, feet, knees, or elbows whenever necessary. This must be thoroughly shaken up each time before using. It is a good, old standby that works. The Rosewater is slightly astringent and healing, while the glycerin acts as a moisturizer.

Chapter XXV

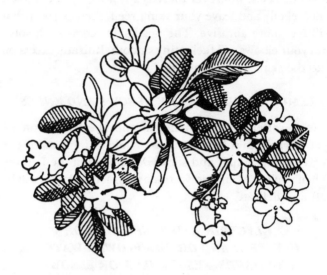

Sun Protectants and Sunning Creams

WHEN IT IS exposed to the sun, the skin produces melanin. And this melanin acts to protect the skin and tans; it also combines with skin protein to protect the skin not only from too much sun, but also from many man-made abuses such as pollution. Unless melanin forms slowly, it will peel off. I remember the first time I went to Hawaii—I have very tough skin and up to that time had never in my life experienced a sunburn. Knowing that I did not burn I went out into the sun on a summer day and stayed all day. That night I was very proud to show off my tan from only one day's exposure to that wonderful Hawaiian sun. My skin never reddened; it was brown immediately, but one week later almost to the day, that poor suntanned skin

356

began to shred in long strips until my suntan had totally disappeared.

Expose yourself to the sun slowly—delicate skin can sometimes take only five minutes' exposure, on each side, on the first day. Skin like mine can take up to an hour on each side on the first day. Change positions frequently on your first few days in the sun and use sun screens if necessary. Wear a hat to protect your hair; if you use tar soap or shampoos they will increase the sun's activity so that 20 minutes of sun is equivalent to about an hour without these aids. Sun bathing in the nude has the added disadvantage of exposing a part of your body to the sun which is generally kept protected—in a woman's case, her breasts, and in a man's, his penis. These are very sensitive and will burn faster than other parts of the body. Fair-skinned people are much more susceptible than darker-skinned people, but even brunettes should use moderation when it comes to sun exposure. In addition, increased contact with the sun heightens one's susceptibility to skin cancer.

Redheads or blonds should use sun screens such as those that contain PABA. They can also take this substance internally (1000 mg. daily), to decrease their sensitivity. If you have herpes, use a substance containing zinc and also take it internally. ". . . Fair skins can also take the oil of unripe Olives in which a small bit of Gum Mastic has been

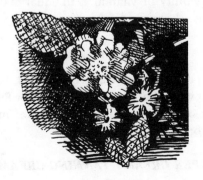

dissolved to preserve the skin from tanning. . . ." This from an old cosmetic herbal.

ART 58

TANNING CREAMS

These creams are easily made; here are some of my favorites:

MAYONNAISE SUN CREAM

Either buy health food mayonnaise or else make your own, and apply to your skin before going out in the sun. Add 1 tablespoon of extra Lemon juice to the mayonnaise to hasten the tan and also an extra protection from the sun.

VITAMIN TAN

Suntanning depletes the body of vitamin C and the B complex, so take more of these essential vitamins when you are spending many hours in the sun. A lack of these vitamins results in patchy, blotchy, or no tan at all.

TANNING CREAM

Mix together equal quantities of Sesame oil and coconut oil, add a quantity of vitamin E to equal 500 units per ounce. Apply whenever necessary.

TAHITIAN TAN

To 1 oz. of Cocoa butter, add 2 oz. coconut oil, 1 oz. Sesame oil, and scent with a few drops of Gardenia or Pikake. This is a favorite of mine and almost duplicates my favorite Monoi oil from Tahiti.

SUPER CREAMY TANNING CREAM

Melt 1 oz. lanolin, add 3 oz. Sesame oil, 2 T. wheat germ oil, and 3 T. Comfrey root water. Beat all together until cold. This is an excellent tanning oil and healing as well.

A AND D OINTMENT

Buy some A and D ointment and soften about 4 oz. over heat. Add 2 oz. Pansy or Violet leaf water and beat together until cold. This ointment is very soothing, softening, and helps to promote an even tan.

SUNBURN COOLERS

These coolers can be made from many different ingredients. The most well known are Cucumber slices applied externally, Potato juice compress, Apple cider vinegar compress, Comfrey leaf water, Marshmallow root water, yogurt diluted with a bit of Lemon juice, baking soda paste, laundry starch paste, black tea as a wash, white of egg beaten with castor oil, or Witch Hazel diluted with glycerin.

SURE-FIRE FIRE COOLER

Take 2 T. *Aloe vera* gel, macerate with 2 T. Comfrey root water and 2 T. castor oil. Add liquid vitamin C, 1 T., and 1 t. vitamin E oil. Mix together until thoroughly blended and apply to the sunburn.

SUNBURN HEALER

The simplest, most effective method of healing a sunburn is to take the leaf of the Aloe, split it down the center and apply this to the sunburn and bind it loosely. Or scoop out the gel, mix with a bit of water for easier spreadability, and simply spread it over the sunburn.

SUNTAN BLEACHERS

Bleachers are needed when your tan is fading, and your

complexion is between that nice warm color of summer and the creamy color of winter. These bleachers include buttermilk, Almond milk, diluted yogurt, diluted Lemon juice, Grape vine juice, Fennel water, White Lily water, Grape juice, or mixtures of these. Apply them as a pack or compress for at least 20 minutes before removing.

LEMON MILK

Soak a couple slices of Lemon in a cup of milk for some hours. Strain out the Lemon and add yogurt to thicken. Apply this cream to your face and body for some hours so that the bleaching action can take effect. Rinse off with a flower water such as Fennel or Elder.

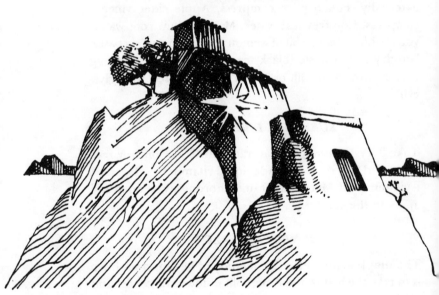

Chapter XXVI

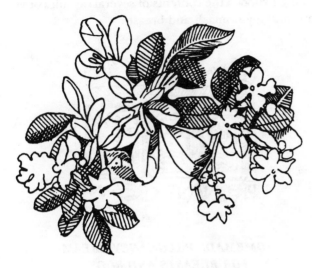

Specials for
the Pregnant Lady

DURING MY RECENT pregnancy I made up and experimented with many different herbal remedies for the common problems of pregnancy. Here are a few of my discoveries:

STOMACH CREAM FOR RAPIDLY STRETCHING SKIN

Make oil of Sage according to directions in Chapter XXII. To 4 oz. of this herbal oil, add 2 oz. of wheat germ oil and 1 oz. of melted lanolin. Beat together until cold.

Stretch marks are very difficult to get rid of (if possible at all) once you've got them. So the trick is to *not* get stretch marks initially rather than try to get rid of them. I used this oil *every night* before going to bed, using enfleurage massage (that is, circular massage starting from the pubic area and working up and around the abdomen). Every single morning I rubbed the contents of several capsules of vitamin E into my stomach and breasts.

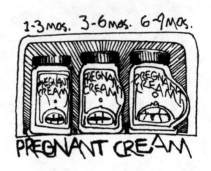

HOMEMADE PREGNANCY CREAM
FOR BREASTS AND BODY

1 oz. Cocoa butter	5 capsules of ADE (providing
4 oz. Olive oil	25,000 units A/oz., 2500
1 oz. hydrous lanolin	units D and 500 units E)
	Absolute oeillet or Carnation
	oil

Melt the Cocoa butter and add the Olive oil and lanolin, beat until mixed, remove from the fire, add the vitamins and the essential oil and beat until cold.

NIPPLE-TOUGHENING CREAM

I wanted to breastfeed my newborn and for the last three months before his birth I massaged my nipples and breasts with a cream made from Comfrey root water and lanolin.

PREGNANCY TEA

Mix together equal quantities of Motherwort, Comfrey

leaf, Ginseng, and Raspberry leaf. Mix the herbs together and drink as many cups a day as you like of this delicious tea.

Raspberry leaf contains fragerine, which eases the pain of childbirth, and acts as a tonic on the uterine muscles. Ginseng is a tonic to the system, Comfrey leaf is a healer, and Motherwort is soothing.

PRENATAL DOUCHE

For that occasional extra heavy but natural vaginal discharge that occurs in the mother-to-be:

> 1 oz. Comfrey root
> 1 oz. Rosemary
> 1 oz. Violet leaf

Pour over these herbs 2 cups of boiling Apple cider vinegar. Infuse for 5 days. Strain out the herbs and douche with 2 T./cup of warm water.

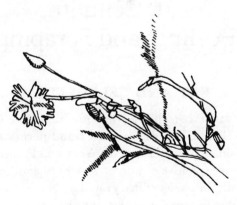

Chapter XXVII

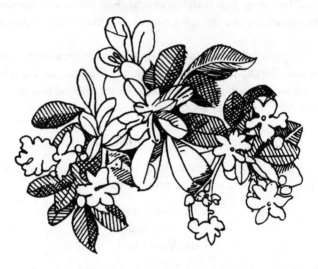

Special Problems:
Fat, Cellulite,
Peeling, and Scraping

FAT AND CELLULITE

WHAT IS CELLULITE (cell-u-leet)? Some reputable doctors say that cellulite, as a disease, is a fraud perpetrated on gullible women by quacks in New York and France. Some feel that it is exploitive of women and is just another word, more exotic, for plain ordinary fat; that there is no alternative for obesity and fat pockets on the body than good old-fashioned diet and supervised exercise. Other physicians, just as reputable, say that cellulite is a gelatinous-like substance, composed of water and waste materials that collects and deposits on the thighs, knees, hips (saddlebag hips), and upper back (dowager's hump), and is caused by imperfect elimination and circulation. Cellulite comes in the soft and hard varieties. Soft cellulite, when pressed, resembles cottage cheese in texture and the hard kind when squeezed is dimpled and pitted like an orange rind.

The anticellulite diet, composed of 4 tiny meals a day, includes fresh ocean fish, raw fruits and vegetables, eggs, unflavored yogurt, lean meat, skim milk, honey, wheat germ, and brewer's yeast. The fruits and vegetables include Grapefruit, Radishes, Pineapples, Onions, Asparagus, Artichokes, Watercress, Sorrel, and Prunes. This diet also includes 8 full glasses of noncarbonated mineral water, which is alkaline and helps to get rid of the body's waste materials. It excludes any processed food or any food that contains artificial colors, flavors, or preservatives.

Exercise is important, especially swimming, bicycle riding, and yoga. Dry skin stimulation with a loofah or friction brush brings blood and therefore nutrients to the surface of the skin and is another form of exercise.

Massage by stroking, scooping, kneading, and rubbing is important to help break down the gel; massage by experts and by the force of water such as ocean waves breaking on the body helps.

Saunas are important because the skin is an organ of excretion; the sauna, by stimulating perspiration, assists in the elimination of these toxic leftovers of food that are deposited in the body as cellulite.

Diuretic herbal teas also assist in the elimination of the waste products and water from the tissues. Herbal teas, yes, but not the chemical diuretics or laxatives which are dangerous and, when taken improperly, are addictive.

Relaxation and proper rest are important for healthy nerves and for those who suffer from poor blood circulation. Here, it is also important to take soothing teas, herbal baths, and oil baths.

This is not a treatise on cellulite but simply a chapter of

recipes to treat it, as well as fat; note these hints would be equally useful for a fat *or* a skinny person.

FAT REMOVAL BY WAXING

1. Dip cheesecloth tapes or strips in warm melted wax[1] and peanut or Olive oil and wrap the strips around the fat areas—such as bottom, hips, thighs, or knees. Lie down with your legs raised for 20 minutes.
2. Remove the strips and then get a good, deep massage using any one of the cellulite massage recipes.
3. Soak muslin tapes or strips in one of the herb solutions that follow and wrap them around the fatty areas. Get into one of the plastic exercise suits and practice your yoga or sit and read or practice breathing.
4. Take a shower, followed by an herbal rinse or take an herbal bath. Since the pores will be open and clean, it is important that you close them either with a cooling astringent or with a cold water rinse. Don't go out for at least an hour.

AVOCADO PIT MASSAGE

Wash any flesh away from the Avocado pit and use it to massage face, throat, chest, or legs. Massage in circular motions everywhere to help break down fat and to firm up flesh. Its also nice to do this massage with an Avocado pit in each hand while you are taking an herb bath. Start at the toes and work up your legs inside and out, in big revolving circles, around the stomach, abdomen, breasts, and on up to the chest, throat, and face. Finish with a stimulating spray from your shower.

[1]Wax will remove hair so add enough oil to moderate this tendency.

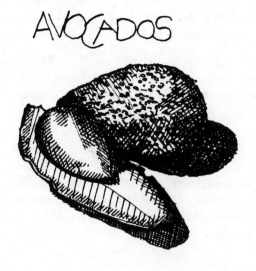

AVOCADOS

CELLULITE MASSAGE OIL

1 oz. Lemon oil
¼ oz. Lime or Grapefruit
    oil

3 oz. vodka and water
    (optional)
       or
3 oz. coconut oil or Al-
    mond oil

Mix the essential oils together. The alcohol (vodka) and the oil (coconut or Almond) function as carrier substances for the essential oils. Mix the essential oils and the carrier substance together and use for massage to facilitate the removal of cellulite.

CELLULITE MASSAGE #2

Mix together 1 oz. essential oil of Lemongrass with 3 oz. of carrier substance as above. Lemongrass is used to improve the circulation of fluids in the tissues and for fluid retention.

CELLULITE MASSAGE #3

1 oz. Sage leaves	1 oz. Marjoram
1 oz. Jaborandi leaves	2 pints brandy

Steep the herbs in the brandy for 2 weeks, shaking the container daily. Strain out the herbs and use them as a poultice or compress. Use the herbed brandy for massage.

CELLULITE MASSAGE #4

Gather the pods from Seaweed that collect on the beach, as fresh as possible. Extract the jelly-like substance from within the pod and have an expert rub this Seapod gel into the skin to help remove cellulite.

EPSOM FAT REMOVAL BATH

Pour 1 lb. Epsom salts into a bath. Make a salt bag of salt in muslin, get in the tub, and while standing rub your whole body down with the salt bag; sit in the tub and soak for 20 minutes. Get out and rub dry with several linen towels, using circular motions.

HERBAL SOAKING SOLUTIONS FOR POULTICE OR COMPRESS

1 oz. Thyme
1 oz. Jaborandi
1 oz. Seaweed

Bring 1 qt. of water and the herbs to a boil, lower the heat and *simmer* for 20 minutes. Strain and use the herbs as a compress on the fat areas and the liquid as a soaking solution for taping (step 3 of Fat Removal) or in a herb bath.

HERBAL SOAK #2

1 sliced Lemon
1 sliced Grapefruit
1 oz. Horsetail

Follow the directions as above.

HERBAL SOAK #3

1 oz. Bladderwrack
1 oz. Dulce
1 oz. Irish moss

This is especially nice as an herbal bath. Follow the directions as listed above.

FOOT AND HAND BATHS FOR CELLULITE

The foot and hand baths as outlined by Maurice Messegué in *Of Men and Plants* include spring Heath flowers, sour Cherry stems, greater Celandine stems and flowers, Couch-grass roots, Broom flowers and young shoots, Corn stigmas, fresh Onion, field Horsetail leaves and Meadowsweet flowers.

DIURETIC TEAS

Beverage teas for fat removal can include the following herbs: Dandelion, Parsley, Alfalfa, Asparagus, Celery, Filaree, Leeks, Mallow stalks, Thyme, Uva ursi, or Pennyroyal.

DIURETIC TEA #2

1 oz. Alfalfa	1 oz. Lemon peel
1 oz. Dandelion	1 oz. Elder
1 oz. Comfrey leaf	1 oz. Camomile

Mix the herbs together and store away in a cool dark place for use. When needed, bring 2 cups of water to a boil and pour over 2 T. or more of the herbs in a preheated non-metal tea pot. Steep for up to 20 minutes. The longer you steep the more potent the brew. Strain and drink throughout the day.

DIURETIC TEA #3

1 oz. Parsley	1 oz. Dulce
1 oz. Sassafras	1 oz. Lemon peel

Mix as above. When drinking the tea, add the juice of ½ Lemon per cup of tea.

SOOTHING TISANE FOR REST AND RELAXATION

1 oz. Violet flowers	1 oz. Linden flowers
1 oz. Camomile flowers	1 oz. Cowslip flowers

Mix as above.

SOOTHING #2

1 oz. Birch leaf
1 oz. Catnip
1 oz. Cherry leaf

Mix as above.

SOOTHING #3

1 oz. Spearmint	1 oz. Red Clover
1 oz. Yerba Buena or	1 oz. Dandelion
Catnip	

Mix as above.

SOOTHING #4

Mix together equal quantities of the following herbs and use as above: Spearmint, Comfrey leaf, Birch leaf, Alfalfa, Lemon Verbena, and Dandelion.

SUPER HERBAL BATH

Mix together equal quantities of the following herbs and use according to the general directions in Chapter XX. Pennyroyal, Lemon peel, Catnip, Strawberry leaf, and Thyme.

OIL BATH

For dry skin and a fat body, the following oils can be added to the bath in a ratio of a few drops oil–¼ oz. of oil per tub full of water: Lemon oil, Grapefruit oil, Lime oil, Lemongrass oil, Lavender oil, Citronella oil, or Sage oil.

PEELING AND SCRAPING

Peeling and scraping the body of its accumulation of oil and perspiration is excellent as a toner for the entire body. In the summer when your skin is extra dry or needs extra lubrication, and in the winter when it is sallow and has been exposed to too much indoor heating, this is an excellent way to revive and refresh the entire system.

THE ROMAN OIL AND SCRAPING BATH

1. Anoint your entire body with either of the following warmed oils: Sage Massage Oil, Pyramid Massage Oil, or Cellulite Massage Oil in Chapter XXII.
2. Exercise in a plastic suit for 10 minutes or without a suit for 20 minutes.
3. Take a 3–10 minute herbal sauna as outlined in Chapter XX.

4. Now scrape your body with a metal or rubber spatula (the Romans called it a strigil). Start with your feet and work up the body, scraping off, rather than pressing in with the spatula. Wipe off the sweat and grime as it accumulates.

5. Now take a warm herbal bath, washing with soap and water and giving yourself a light scrub down with a friction mitt or loofah.

6. Close the pores with a cool rinsing or if you can stand it a cold shower.

7. If your body has especially dry skin you may wish another anointing of light oil or an aroma massage. You will feel wonderful and clean—all pink and shiny.

MORE PEELING TECHNIQUES

The Super Cleansing Bath in Chapter XX (Epsom salts and salt) is excellent as a means of exfoliating, peeling off, the outer, dead, flaky layer of the skin. Other ways to get rid of this are by bathing and scrubbing with a Cornmeal bag or any of these: scrubbing with a hemp or horsehair friction strap or a loofah; a gritty mixture of ground Papaya seeds and Papaya flesh; a mashed half of Avocado mixed with a half cup of salt; rubbing the meaty rather than juicy slices of Tomato all over your body; or scrubbing with soap and a bristle bath brush. All of these are to be followed by a soap and water bath or shower and a cooling rinse.

Part III

THE EXTRA-SPECIAL MAKE-YOUR-BODY-FEEL-GOOD DAY

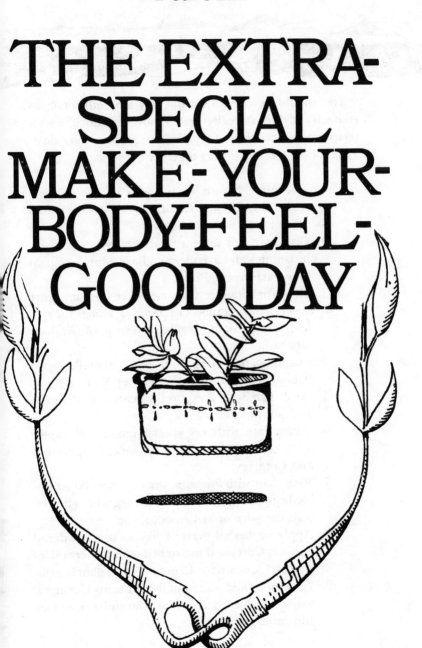

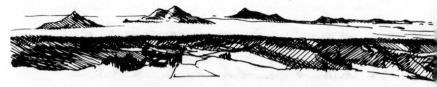

You should devote at least one day a month totally to yourself. It doesn't really matter how you do it, which recipe you use, or if you follow my suggestions—just do it. This is how I keep "my act together."

1. The night before wrap hands in honey, eggs, Almond meal, and Comfrey root. Cover with a pair of long white kid gloves.
2. Give hair and scalp a treatment by a thorough brushing with Lavender and Basil oil and wrap up in a scarf overnight.
3. Sleep for a long restful time, wake up, eat yogurt and my own granola (see *Herbs & Things* for recipe), read the paper, have a cup of Arabian mocha.
4. Shampoo hair once with any herbal shampoo (Chapter XV) and rinse (Chapter XVI).
5. Wash hair with 2 egg yolks beaten until frothy and put on a shower cap.
6. Steam face with my special mixture (Chapter VII), or with Lavender, Camomile, Peppermint, and Comfrey.
7. Rinse hair with *lukewarm water* (please, no scrambled eggs), and wash again with egg whites beaten with the juice of ½ Lemon. Rinse.
8. Apply an herbal mask; I like to use powdered Pansies, Cornmeal moistened with buttermilk or yogurt. Lie down for 15 minutes on a slant board.
9. Take a soap and water hot shower using Cornmeal soap and a loofah as a scrub. Carefully rinse hair and mask off of face.

10. Jump instantly into a hot herbal bath (I like to use the Ginseng Bath, Chapter XX). Rub down lightly with a salt bag (spray a bit of Lavender or Basil on the salt). Condition your heels with pumice and your elbows with Avocado peel. Start your manicure and pedicure by pushing down your softened cuticles with an orange stick.

11. Apply the Honey Pat but don't pat, or apply an Orange Jelly mask made of Orange juice and Quince.

12. Rinse with warm water and then with cool water or if you can stand it, take a cold shower.

13. Wrap in a giant towel and air dry.

14. Finish your manicure and pedicure.

15. Finish up with a soothing aroma-massage (I like to use Spanish Jasmine as a base with Safflower and wheat germ).

16. Brush your hair from top to bottom.

Now I feel like a new woman, all pink and shiny and ready for the next exhausting and invigorating month.

THE EXTRA-SPECIAL
HERBAL HANDSOME TIME FOR MEN

Men shouldn't neglect their bodies for it is certainly not feminizing to strive to be clean and healthy. My husband doesn't spend an entire day cleaning and beautifying himself; it only takes an hour, but he does it much more often than I. Here is his regime:

1. Facial steam of Licorice, Comfrey, and Rosemary.

2. Get into a hot herbal bath of anything that happens to be on hand.

3. Apply Apri-Honey (Chapter XIV) and soak and read for an hour or more, continually adding a

small stream of hot water. I occasionally give him a minimanicure and pedicure.

4. He shaves with soap, either Black Forest Herbal or Neca 7, and scrubs with the soap, water, and a loofah.
5. A warm rinse with fresh water is followed by a cold rinse.
6. Wrap in an enormous towel, stalk around the house like a giant pear on stalks, and air dry.

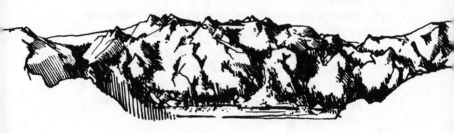

Part IV

COSMETICS USED IN MAGIC

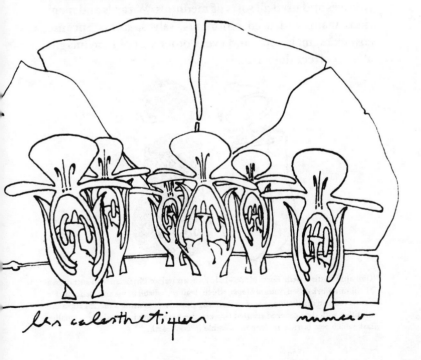

les caltesthetiques   numero

Witch is a word derived from "wica" or "wise ones." And the witches, philosophers, magicians, alchemists of ancient times believed that one's ability in magic was merely the possession of a perfect knowledge of natural things. This knowledge encompassed all aspects of life: knowing the natural vibration of minerals and metals and how they vibrated to color; how color, scent, and sound were analogous; knowing vibrations of *plants* and use of this knowledge for one's own purpose. Giovanni Battista della Porta[1] said that it behooved the Magician to be a perfect Philosopher, to be a skillful Physician and skilled Physic, to be a Master Herbalist, and to excell at Mathematics, especially Astrology. The science of magic was in fact regarded as the art or skill of worshipping God, and is so to this day, though it is obscured (but undiminished) by the more organized "religions."

This science manifested itself in many forms and all cultures and used all sorts of mediums. Wizards and magicians made and used ointments, salves, scents, incense, cosmetics, make-ups, and every other sort of item imaginable to effect their rituals.

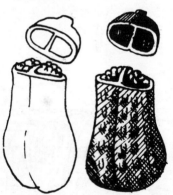

[1]Giovanni Battista della Porta (1538–1615) was an Italian Physician who authored a 20-volume work called *Natural Magic*, which dealt with distillations and alchemy. He discovered sun distillation, a way of distilling fine essences using a matras set in the sun filled with dew-covered scented flowers, the neck being inserted into a smaller flask which was buried as deep as possible in cool earth.

Wizards' Ointments had a very early origin. In ancient times, Chaldean priests, Arabian chemists and magicians of every sort compounded oils for specific magical uses. These contained aromatics and fragrant aromata consecrated to Gods of one sort and another. Oils and ointments have seen usage throughout history, as oils and perfumes have played an important part in evocatory magic. Witches rubbed them upon witches to induce visionary and trance states while drugging the senses; and they were rubbed on the victim to create a state of total drugged obedience. These ointments were often given to or rubbed on the unwary as cosmetic gifts. Magicians and wizards of ancient times were accustomed to rubbing their bodies with oils and ointments and even today this is a way of getting in touch with the supernatural to bring about states of ecstasy. In Castaneda's *The Teachings of Don Juan* the sorcerer gets in touch with Power by rubbing himself with the herb as an oil. In this instance he uses Datura which he describes as very poisonous and accessible to few sorcerers. In other cases the herbs Hemlock or Aconite made into ointments were rubbed on the body as a prelude to performing witchcraft; these altered perception drastically. There are many ointments listed in magical literature:

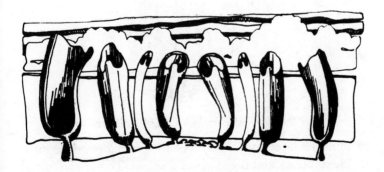

OILS AND OINTMENTS

WITCH OINTMENT

An unknown herb and grease from an animal were mixed into an ointment which was rubbed on a staff. With this the Irish witch was able to fly and gallop about through any kind of weather.

—*Witchcraft Facts*

TO RENDER A VICTIM HELPLESS

A witch will use Belladonna in her rubbing ointments when making a love potion.

TO REDUCE THE ARDOUR OF LOVE
(i.e., Reduce the Size of an Erection)

Make a poultice or ointment of Hemlock and apply this to the afflicted member.

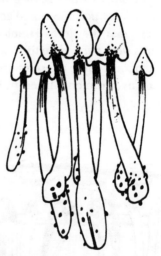

TO PROVOKE A MAN TO VENERY

Anoint the large toe of his right foot with a cosmetic oil made of honey and the ashes of a weasel. To increase the efficaciousness of this magical ointment add the herbs of sexual love and desire such as the Coriander, the Jasmine and the Violet that have been picked in the last quarter of the moon.

TO GO TO A SABBATH

Witches had to prepare ointments made of herbs and animal matter. This ointment enabled the witch to use levitation, to fly about on her broom and to become invisible. Many herbs were used in these ointments, mainly the poisonous herbs such as the herbs of Saturn—Wolfbane, Hellebore, Henbane, Hemlock, Hemp, Nightshade, but also other herbs with magical reputations such as Parsley, Vervain, or Rue. The ointment had to be carefully smeared upon the whole body but especially upon the forehead and in the armpits. (See *Herbs & Things*, pp. 259 and 260, "For Riding on a Broomstick and Flying.")

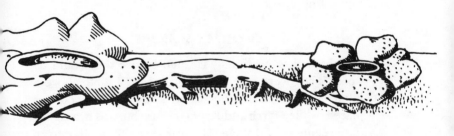

INVISIBILITY HERBS

There were many of these herbs used to create ointments which when rubbed on the maker of the ointment gave invisibility. But it was also important to wear the ring of invisibility and carry the Heliotrope. The herbs used in these ointments were Lungwort, Nightshade, Speedwell and others.

DEATH OINTMENTS

These ointments also have an old and justifiably fearsome reputation. One said to come from an Egyptian papyrus on magic features rubbing a man with an ointment made of cooked 2-tailed lizard.

LYCANTHROPY

Ointments made of Saturnic herbs were said to change people into beasts. One such happening is recorded in France in 1521 where it was stated in a murder trial that a man named Michael had made an ointment that turned him into a wolf when he rubbed himself with it. He described how he behaved and had mauled and killed many adults and children while a wolf. Belladonna and deadly Nightshade were used in such ointments, obviously to interesting effect.

EGYPTIAN SCARABS

Scarabs had to be ritually cleaned before they could be worn. They were carved and placed on a table above a linen cloth. Beneath the scarab some Olive wood was placed, while Myrrh and Kyphi incense burned in a censer in the center of the table. The scarab was then put into an ointment of Lilies, Cinnamon, or Myrrh and left for 3 days followed by a celebration and sacrifice during which the ring was removed from the ointment and ". . . anoint thyself with the unction from it. Thou shalt anoint thyself early in the morning . . . and pronounce the words in this spell, 'I am Thoth, the inventor and founder of medicines and letters; come to me, thou that art under the earth, rise up to me, thou great spirit'."

—*Egyptian Magic* by E. A. Wallis Budge, p. 42.

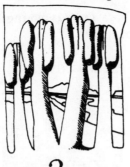

2
EGYPTIAN OINTMENTS

They were often composed of cedar oil. These along with incense, magical pictures, spells and formulas were all used to assist the soul into the next world. ". . . Among the objects presented to the deceased in these ceremonies scents and perfumed unguents play a prominent part. . . . To certain kinds of oil, magical properties have been attached from time immemorial in the East, and the important place which they occupied in the ceremonies and rituals of many nations proves that remarkable effects are expected to follow their use. The living made use of oil to soften the skin and to preserve it from the parching heat of the sun, and the dead were anointed with it during the process of mummification so that their skins might, through the magical words which were pronounced whilst it was being rubbed on them, remain soft for all time, and so that the curative properties of the oil might heal the wounds which the mummifiers had made. . . ."

—*Egyptian Magic* by E. A. Wallis Budge, pp. 203 and 204

Oil appears in many Egyptian prescriptions and with its magical properties, transformations could be accomplished. It was useful to the physician for its healing qualities and to the magician for its magical qualities. In *Egyptian Magic,* a woman is described as becoming transformed into a night raven by anointing herself with oil and uttering a magical spell.

MAKE-UPS AND COSMETIC WATERS

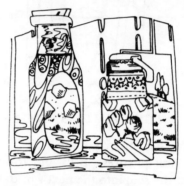

Aqua Toffana Aquetta di Napoli was a poisonous water invented by the notorious female poisoner, Teofania di Adamo, aka Torfano. She started her shady business in the city of Palermo in 1650, moved to Naples and there fashioned the poisonous water (or unguent) that bore her name. It is said that with this water she poisoned over 600 persons. The liquid was made of hogs lard and arsenic or a water of arsenic. And it was drunk, applied externally as a cosmetic, or the ointment was applied or added to foods. Torfano escaped suspicion for years because at that time in Naples a holy water of the same name was also being circulated.

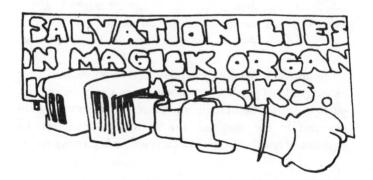

BELLADONNA EYEWASH

This eyewash was used by Italian ladies to enlarge the pupil of their eye making them more luminous and therefore more attractive.

TO ENCOURAGE SENSUALITY

A water is made of the Myrtle leaf and rubbed all over the body. You can also take a bath in great quantities of the herb or use it in all your creams and salves.

—Legends of Herb Magic

GOOD INFLUENCE SEED RUB

If someone is a bad influence (and I can see where this rub might be of enormous value to parents whose friends have "bad" kids) rub the root of the Celery on that person and great changes will occur.

—Legends of Herb Magic

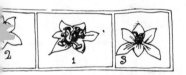 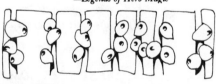

LOVING BATH HERBS

Loving Bath Herbs can be made with a mixture of Sandalwood, Orris root, and Myrrh. This is said to have a calming and quieting effect on any person the bather might come into contact with.

—An Ancient Book of Formulas

MAGIC ATTRACTING POWDER

This powder can be made with Orris root powder. Sprinkle it all over yourself and rub it carefully into the skin. This is said to attract the love of one of the opposite sex.

—Legends of Herb Magic

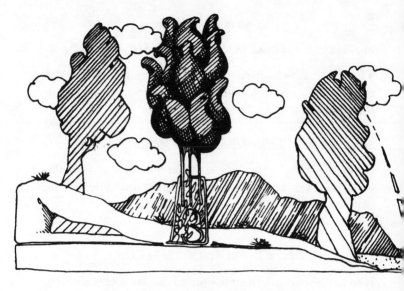

LOVE IN IDLENESS (PANSIES)

Fetch me that flower; the herb I shew'd thee once:
The juice of it on sleeping eyelids laid
Will make a man or woman madly dote
Upon the next live creature that it sees.

—*Shakespeare (Oberon to Puck)*

BEET TOPS COMPLEXION WATERS

These waters are used in the Ozarks to give a pink color to the skin but a girl who uses such a thing and is praised for her pretty complexion will not share her cosmetic secrets because she considers them a charm and, if spoken of, the spell would be broken and then the cosmetic would not work. ***Chicken hearts*** if eaten RAW are said to make any girl pretty. There are other charms and spells connected with beauty: touch your face to a ***Dead man's hand*** to discourage pimples, blackheads, large pores, or other complexion marks; cure chapped lips by ***kissing*** the middle-bar of a split rail fence; ***Urine*** treatments will cure falling hair; cut your hair during the ***new moon*** to encourage luxuriant growth; combing ***wet hair*** will make it coarse (of course combing wet hair stretches it out and causes it to break easily and be less elastic). There are many many more charms and spells in *Ozark Magic and Folklore* by Vance Randolph.

FOOT BATHS

Foot baths of herbs were used to induce sleep and herbs were used to both help and hinder a witch.

> *"Trefoil, vervain, John's wort, dill,*
> *Hinder witches of their will."*

DRAGON'S BLOOD

This was once thought to be real dragon's blood but is actually the resin from the fruit of the dragon tree and has a long history of medical and magical usage. Now it is used only occasionally in cosmetics or love charms. See p. 143 See p. 143 *Herbs & Things*.

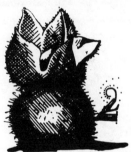

HENBANE

This is a poisonous herb used in magic and also as a depilatory: the Henbane seed is mixed with ant eggs and all is reduced to a fine powder to be applied to the hairy spot twice a day, but I certainly do not recommend its use.

KOHL

A cosmetic used in the East, Kohl is often contaminated

with lead and has been implicated in many cases of eye disease and blindness. It is said that long term use of Kohl will cause madness (as a result of lead poisoning?). This cosmetic is painted around the eye to make it appear larger and darker. It has been mentioned in Egyptian papyrus, as well as Eastern and Roman works.

HEMP LOTION

This lotion is made by infusing the young plants in water for 24 hours and then combing the hair with it. It is said that the combing done along with certain verbal spells (!) will cause the hair to grow long and strong.

ARTFUL ARSENIC EYES

In other days an eye make-up was made of seven parts of Lime mixed with three of orpiment (a mineral containing arsenic). This was used by Turkish women as an eye paint and also as a depilatory (!).

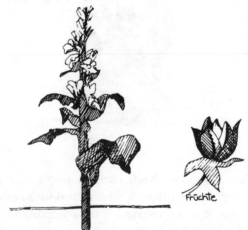

SCENTS, PERFUMES, INCENSE

It has long been known that odors have a curious effect upon man and animal. They affect both the natural and supernatural worlds and their usage as psychological stimulants is certainly well established. Incense has been employed in religious ceremonies and is considered food for the Gods; perfumes are used as aphrodisiacs and in love potions. To every Spirit, every Angel, good or bad, a characteristic and appropriate odor has been assigned. Scented candles of the appropriate odor are used in magical ceremonies to aid the spell, scented baths of essences and herbs are used not only to soothe the skin but to scent it and render it acceptable to the proper spirit; or to entice lovers or the spirit as a lover. Perfumes and fumigations play an important part in ritual and magical evocations. Usually the strong and foul smelling herbs are reserved for the demons, Henbane with its distinct cat's urine smell, musty Mullein, Dog Fennel that grows in empty lots and often smells foul and dirtied, or the strong green sick smell of the Foxglove.

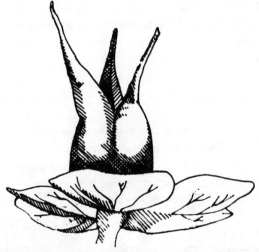

THE ART OF POISON was practiced by the de Medicis who were skilled in using all manner of tools, rings, gloves, or cosmetics as the poison vehicle. Catherine de Médicis trained her perfumer in this nefarious art of killing persons either through inhalation of sweetly scented perfumes or by absorption through the skin from poisoned gloves or rings (this is certainly an interesting form of aromatherapy).

CLEOPATRA INCENSE

It is said in a book of magic that Cleopatra saturated her body and her clothes in the fumes of incense so that her feminine wiles would be greatly increased and she could make slaves of men. Her incense was composed of 8 oz. Winter's Bark, 12 oz. Sandalwood, 4 oz. each of Orris root, Patchouli, Myrrh, Frankincense, and a Wood Base and 2 oz. of Saltpeter to make the incense sparkle when burned. She seemed to do pretty well with it too.

My father was a man with a green thumb; Grapes thrived under his care and Rosemary was his herb. He did not believe in magic but he certainly believed in herbs. He died last year and Shakespeare wrote words hundreds of years ago that seem to me to make a fitting part of this book.

A SPECIAL DEDICATION TO MY FATHER

> *. . . I would give you some violets, but they withered all when my father died.*

—*Shakespeare (Ophelia speaking)*

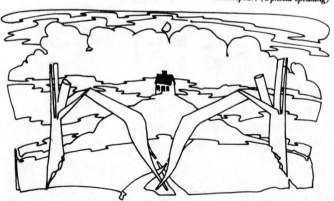

A SELECTED BIBLIOGRAPHY

This part was fittingly completed on All Hallow's Eve, October 31, 1975. My research here was immensely helped by the following books: *The Magic of Herbs* by Mrs. C. F. Leyel; *The Story of Alchemy and Early Chemistry* by John M. Stillman; *Gypsy Sorcery and Fortune-Telling* by Charles Godfrey Leland; *Ozark Magic and Folklore* by Vance Randolph; *Legends of Herb & Oil Magic* by Lewis de Claremont; *The Ancient Book of Formulas* published by Dorene Publ. Dallas, Texas; *A Treasury of Witchcraft* by Harry E. Wedeck; *Witches and Their Craft* by Ronald Seth; *Mastering Witchcraft* by Paul Huson; *Egyptian Magic* by E. A. Wallis Budge; *The Gods of the Egyptians* by E. A. Wallis Budge; *A Garden of Herbs* by E. S. Rohde; *Witchcraft, Magic & Alchemy* by Grillot de Givry.

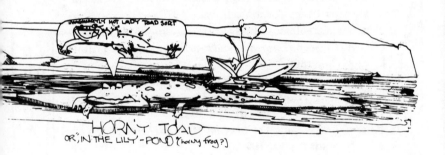

HORN'Y TOAD
OR, IN THE LILY-POND (horny frog?)

Bibliography

Adamson, Helen Lyon, *Grandmother's Household Hints*. New York, Paperback Library, Inc., 1963.

Brown, Alice Cooke, *Early American Herb Recipes*. New York, Bonanza Books, 1966.

Buchman, Dian Dincin, *Feed Your Face*. London, Duckworth, 1973.

Clark, Linda, *Secrets of Health and Beauty*. New York, Pyramid Books, 1969.

Culpeper's English Physician; and Complete Herbal, 15th edition. London, W. Lewis, St. John's Square, 1813.

Davis, Adelle, *Let's Eat Right to Keep Fit*. New York, Harcourt Brace Jovanovich, Inc., 1970.

Dussauce, Professor H., *A General Treatise on the Manufacture of Soap, Theoretical and Practical*. London, Trubner & Co., 1869.

Freeman, Margaret B., *Herbs for the Mediaeval Household for Cooking, Healing and Divers Uses*. New York, The Metropolitan Museum of Art, 1943.

Glenn, Lucie, *Cosmetics You Can Make at Home*. New York, Bantam Books, 1972.

Grieve, M., *A Modern Herbal*. 2 vols., New York, Hafner Publishing Company, 1971 (1931).

Heritage, Ford, *Composition and Facts About Foods*. Woodstown, New Jersey, Ford Heritage, 1968.

Hewitt, James, *Facial Isometrics for Youth and Beauty*. New York, Award Books, 1970.

Home Dissertations: an Offering to the Household For Economical and Practical Skill in Cookery, Orderly Domestic Management, and Nicety in the Appointments of Home. Excerpts from Favorite Authors, 2nd edition. San Francisco, Goldberg, Bowen and Lebenbaum, Publ., 1891.

Housekeeping in Old Virginia, edited by Marion Cabell Tyree. Louisville, John P. Morton and Company, 1879.

Keller, Jeanne, *Healing with Water: Special Applications and Uses of Water in Home Remedies for Everyday Ailments.* West Nyack, New York, Parker Publishing Co., 1968.

Kneipp, Sebastan, *My Water-cure.* Bavaria, Jos. Koesel, 1956 (1886).

Kunin, Matilda and Patricia Swig, *A San Francisco Little Black Book of Beauty.* San Francisco, 1972.

Lawson, Donna, *Mother Nature's Beauty Cupboard.* New York, Thomas Y. Crowell Company, 1973.

Leyel, Mrs. C. F., *Herbal Delights.* London, Faber and Faber Limited, 1937.

————, *The Magic of Herbs.* New York, Harcourt, Brace & Company, 1926.

Maxwell, Cathleen, *The Claverton Herbal.* Somerset, England, The American Museum, 1972.

Melendy, Mary Ries, *Vivilore: The Pathway to Mental and Physical Perfection.* Chicago, W. R. Vansant, 1904.

Messegué, Maurice, *Of Men and Plants.* New York, The Macmillan Company, 1973.

Meyer, Joseph E., *The Herbalist.* Hammond, Indiana, Indiana Botanical Gardens, 1932.

Northcote, Lady Rosalind, *The Book of Herbs.* London and New York, John Lane: The Bodley Head, 1903.

Pierce, R. V., *The People's Common Sense Medical Adviser in Plain English: or, Medicine Simplified.* New York, World's Dispensary Printing Office and Bindery, 1895.

Plat, Sir Hugh, *Delightes for Ladies.* London, England, 1602. (reprinted from the edition of 1627, illustrations from 1609 edition). Collated and edited by Violet and Hal W. Trovillion in 1939.

Present Knowledge in Nutrition, 3rd edition. New York, The Nutrition Foundation, Inc., 1967.

Pugh, Katie, *Hair thru Diet.* Virginia, Graphic Arts Press, 1970 (1961).

Romanne-James, C., *Herb-Lore for Housewives.* London, Herbert Jenkins Ltd., 1938.

Rose, Jeanne, *Herbs & Things: Jeanne Rose's Herbal*. New York, Grosset & Dunlap, 1972.

Roth, Beulah, *The Fresh Avocado Beauty Book*. California, The Avocado Growers, 1972.

————, *The International Beauty Book*. Los Angeles, California, Price/Stern/Sloan, 1970.

Stabile, Toni, *Cosmetics Trick or Treat*. New York, ARC Books, 1970.

Szekely, Edmond Bordeaux, *The Golden Door Book of Beauty and Health*. Los Angeles, The Ward Ritchie Press, 1967.

————, *Healing Waters*. San Diego, Academy Books, 1973.

Thomas, Virginia Castleton, *My Secrets of Natural Beauty*. New Canaan, Conn., 1972.

Thomson, James C. and C. Leslie Thomson, *Healthy Hair*. New York, ARC Books, 1970.

The Toilet of Flora; or, A Collection of the Most Simple and Approved Methods of Preparing. . . ., reprinted from the edition dated 1779, London, J. Murray.

Tromovitch, Theodore A., *Acne: Its Causes and Control*. San Francisco, California, 1966.

Tromovitch, Theodore A. and Donald M. Kay, *Atopic Dermatitis: Its Causes and Control*. San Francisco, California, 1970.

————, *Psoriasis: Its Causes and Control*. San Francisco, California, 1967.

————, *Skin Cancer: Its Causes and Control*. San Francisco, California, 1969.

Vogel, Virgil J., *American Indian Medicine*. Oklahoma, University of Oklahoma Press, 1970.

Winter, Ruth, *A Consumer's Dictionary of Cosmetic Ingredients*. New York, Crown Publishers, Inc., 1974.

Wren, R. C., *Potter's New Encyclopedia of Botanical Drugs and Preparations*. Sussex, England, Health Science Press, 1968. (First published, 1939.)

Yaller, Robert and Raye, *The Health Spas*. Santa Barbara, Woodbridge Press Publishing Co., 1974.

Index

(The page numbers in boldface after each plant or herb entry indicate where a detailed description of the plant or herb may be found.)